mBook: Making Masking Manageable

Preliminary Edition

Teri A Hamill, PhD

audstudent.com
and Professor,
Nova Southeastern University
Ft Lauderdale, FL

www.audstudent.com
available in hardcopy from Amazon.com

Copyright 2016.

All rights reserved.

May not be reproduced without permission.

Cover art utilizes images from Design by Freepik.com

http:freepik.com

ISBN-13: 978-1537040080
ISBN-10: 1537040081

Disclaimer

The author believes the information to be correct, but neither the author, audstudent.com, nor the publisher is liable for errors within the text. The professional must use appropriate clinical judgment and ensure that he or she is performing testing competently and appropriately. We make no warranty of the information and are not responsible for the consequences of any errors or incomplete information.

Acknowledgements; Our Philosophy, and a Rant; Games!!

Acknowledgments

My NSU students are thanked beyond belief for their comments, suggestions and edits along the way.

My husband, Tom Barron, inspired all this. He is the engineering brains beyond audstudent.com. He told me that the audstudent.com pages that get the most hits are related to masking, even though they are marginal quality web 1.0 pages. We worked together to utilize technology to make this challenging subject more manageable. (Tom: can we go sailing now?)

Philosophy / Rant

Will an alternative, lower-cost, learning system work? Can we save students money? Can we make learning easier and more fun?

When a professor writes a book, like this one, if the publisher agrees to take on the project, who makes $$?

- Your university bookstore / online retailer
- The publisher
- The company that printed the book
- The book shipper
- The author receives 10% of what the bookstore / retailer bought the book for (note: not what YOU paid)

Who pays for all this?

- The student

Meanwhile, the professor has agreed never again to use the words or figures other than what is published, even if the book doesn't sell well.

Let's try another model.

- Want the e-book? Free. Very green! Currently included with the game apps.
- Want a hardcopy? Are you sure? OK, I too like to highlight, write in the margins, … You need to pay us (a buck or two, it took work to get all this into print format), and you need to pay Amazon (whatever they say it costs; they tabulate the final cost.)
- GAMES!!! This is the real advancement. So, let's make that a new heading.

Games and Assignments

You attend class presentations, you read, you do homework/quizzes, and you get feedback. Assignment/test feedback is (eventually) great, but there is a better way! eBook chapter 4 and mQuest games let you know if you "get it".

- Games = instant feedback
- Games = integrated with your readings
- We hope professors will give parallel assignments. (Accessed by going to www.audstudent.com, then select resources.) It's easier to study from hardcopy assignments than just web and game stuff.

One disadvantage to not using a commercial publisher is that we don't have their professional editors. That means errors leak through. (They do even when you publish with a commercial firm). If – heck, when!!! – you find errors, would you be so kind as to let us know? Submit feedback to audstudent.com@gmail.com.

Contents

Chapter 1 An Analogy for Beginners; Abbreviations, Definitions, and Rules; Formulae Quick Reference Summaries 1

Chapter 2 When Masking is Needed for Air-Conduction Testing 17

Chapter 3 When to Mask for Bone-Conduction Testing 27

Chapter 4 Recognizing the Need for Masking 33

Chapter 5 Plateau Masking for Air-Conduction Testing 45

Chapter 6 Plateau Masking for Bone-Conduction Testing 63

Chapter 7 What is Formula Masking and Why Use It? 83

Chapter 8 Formula Masking for Pure-Tone Air-Conduction Testing 87

Chapter 9 Formula Masking for Pure-Tone Bone-Conduction Testing 99

Chapter 10 Formula Masking for Speech Stimuli 129

Chapter 1

An Analogy for Beginners; Abbreviations, Definitions, and Rules; Formulae Quick Reference Summaries

Starting on page 10 is a reference guide for those who want to quickly access a formula, or need a reminder of what the many abbreviations stand for in this e-book or the associated games.

For first time readers, there is an analogy that may be of interest, but after that, the remainder is quick references for those who have already completed the book, so you would then skip to Chapter 2

Introduction and an Analogy

Masking is one of the more challenging topics for first year audiology students. There are some fundamental concepts of crossover and crossback that have to be understood. Perhaps an analogy will help. Perhaps not, but it probably won't hurt, so let's try.

Sarah, age 3, is in the kitchen with her father who is keeping her busy making cookies. Sarah's mother is in the next room, behind a closed door, talking to Sarah's grandmother who wants to know what to buy Sarah for her upcoming birthday.

Conversation Overheard

Uh oh! Sarah's father can hear bits of the phone conversation from the other room; the "what to get Sarah" conversation has "crossed over" to the kitchen, which means risk that Sarah's birthday gift won't be a surprise.

Masking Crossover

In hearing testing, some of the test ear signal can spill over to the non-test ear. Just as we want only the grandmother to hear the birthday gift suggestions, not Sarah, we want only the test ear to hear the tone (or speech testing material). We don't want the response to come from the non-test ear. When the sound is conveyed from the test ear to the non-test ear, it is said to have "crossed over".

Masking During Cookie Making

Sarah's father quickly turns on some music, which is louder than the faint murmur of the conversation in the other room. He has masked the "crossover".

Masking During Masking

To prevent the non-test ear from detecting the crossed-over tone, noise will be put into the non-test ear.

Insufficient Masking

Sarah complains that she doesn't like that song and changes it, alas to one that is quieter. Dad can hear bits of the conversation, so he asks Sarah to turn up the volume.

Chapter 1. Analogy

Undermasking

Just putting some noise in the non-test ear doesn't mean it's enough noise. We will consider if we may be undermasking.

Crossback – the Radio is Audible in the Room Next Door

Not unexpectedly, the radio may be heard in the room where grandmother and mother are talking by phone. If the radio is lower than the conversation, it's not a problem.

Crossback in Masking

In masking, if the noise that is meant to keep the non-test ear from hearing the test ear tone is loud enough, it can cross back to the test ear cochlea. If some of the masking noise sent to the non-test ear sneaks over to the test ear, that's not necessarily a problem. As long as the crossed back noise is less intense than the signal level (reaching the test ear cochlea), then it won't alter the test results.

Crossback Interfering with (Masking) the Phone Conversation

A favorite song comes on and Sarah turns up the volume considerably and stops her cookie making to dance to the music. The grandmother complains "Can you turn down the radio you have in the background? It's louder than you are and I'm having trouble understanding you." Problematically, Sarah's tunes have crossed from the kitchen back to the room where the all-important conversation about gift choices is taking place.

Overmasking

When the masking noise interferes with hearing of the test ear signal, then "crossback" is "overmasking". (We want to mask -- prevent the hearing of the crossover -- but we don't want so much masking that it crosses back to the test ear and interferes with hearing of the signal in the test ear.) Sometimes the solution is to turn down the masker noise.

I'll Have to Phone You Later!

But what if the mother's cell phone was lousy and/or the grandmother's phone had low volume and the only way for them to converse is if the mother speaks very loudly? The mother's loud voice reaches the kitchen, so the father has to have the radio that loud to keep Sarah from hearing. This is a no-win situation. The radio is interfering with the phone conversation, so Grandmother can't hear Sarah's mother, but the mother needs to speak loudly.

Masking Dilemmas

Sometimes we need a lot of masking noise to mask the crossover, but that crosses back and keeps the test ear from hearing the tone. If adjustments cannot be made to prevent audible crossover (keeps non-test ear from hearing) without having the confounding problem of cross back causing overmasking (noise interfering with test ear hearing), then that is called a masking dilemma. It's only a dilemma if there is no solution. If you have to work at adjusting the noise level but can find a level that works, then it's not a true dilemma.

Chapter 1. Analogy

Not All Doors Are Created Equal

Sarah's mother wouldn't have much luck at keeping the phone conversation secret if a glass bead curtain separated the two rooms – the decorative curtain provides no sound attenuation. (Sarah's mother would have known that other sound needs to mask her conversation right from the start.) The hollow-core interior doors in most homes provide pretty minimal sound attenuation; if the door is solid wood, the attenuation would be better.

Different Transducers Have Different Interaural Attenuation Values

Attenuation is a loss of sound – the glass curtain offered no attenuation. In audiologic testing we are concerned with the between-ears attenuation, which is termed the interaural attenuation.

Bone vibrators are the glass curtain of the audiology world. If you put the oscillator on the right ear, the bones of the head are all vibrating together and you send the entire signal over to the left ear.

Supra-aural earphones are akin to the hollow-core door. Insert earphones have the best interaural attenuation – they convey the least sound from test ear to non-test ear, or noise from non-test ear back to the test ear.

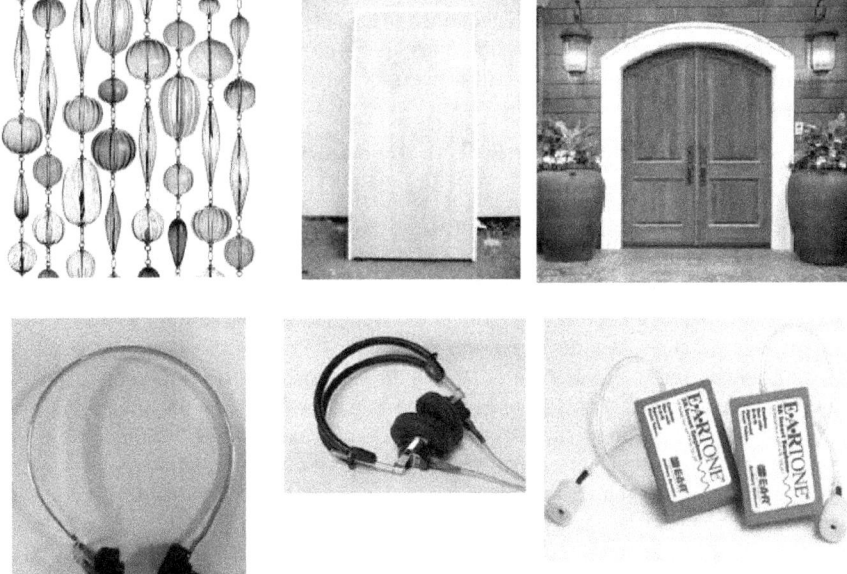

Figure 1-1. Lower panel. Bone oscillator (left) testing has no interaural attenuation, supra-aural earphones, such as this TDH-50P style shown at center, offer modest interaural attenuation. The earphone with the best (greatest) interaural attenuation is the insert earphone (right).

Chapter 1. Analogy

The Home with Only Glass Bead Interior Doors

Let's imagine that Sarah's parents are "new-age" types who believe that family should not be separated by solid doors. And since it's raining outside, the mother is not inclined to go outside to make the phone call. Mom will be easily heard, any music that is in the kitchen will readily cross back to Mom and interfere with the Grandmother's hearing about what gifts Sarah would like.

Solution: have Sarah wear earphones to listen to the music while baking the cookies. Now, for this analogy to work, the earphones have to be the foam type that sit on top of the ear and don't block sound out – they just present the music directly to Sarah, which allows masking. Sarah's wearing of earphones has the advantage of less chance of cross-back. Imagine how loud the music presented via earphones would have to be to be heard by Grandmother.

When Testing via Bone-Conduction, Present the Masking with Earphones

Since bone-conducted sound all crosses to the non-test ear, we have an inherent problem. The non-test ear is always stimulated. If you were to try to put masking noise into the non-test ear by bone conduction, it would cross right back and overmask. The solution is to put the masking noise in by air-conduction – using an insert earphone or supra-aural earphone. The insert earphones are not preventing the crossover, they are not creating any attenuation (just as the foam earphones sitting in Sarah's conchas would not mask her mother's conversation if the music is off). It just means that we can mask (Sarah won't hear) – and the noise won't immediately overmask (won't interfere with the phone conversation).

Sarah and Her Father Potentially Hear Mom Better than Grandmother Does

This part of the analogy is a bit weak, but let's try it. Could there ever be a time when the mother's voice (through the glass curtain) is more audible in the kitchen than over the phone? Sure, how about if phone Grandmother was using had insufficient volume? Well, that doesn't make for a good analogy for bone-conduction testing, so we are going to have to create a far-fetched scenario. I'll have to make Sarah an official Hamill for a moment, though I have no such niece. Hamills don't give the extended family real Christmas gifts, we exchange gag gifts. The person who gives the best gag gift wins the coveted fish slippers, which are … slippers shaped like fish. The winner displays the fish slippers but never wears them, as they must be surrendered to the next year's winner without toe jam contamination. Sarah's Aunt Mary gave Sarah a pair of earphones that have giant dog ears attached, as shown in Figure 1-2. Now Sarah can hear sounds better than average so long as she's looking in that direction of the sound source, and the cookie-cutting Sarah is indeed looking at the glass beaded door, wondering who her mother is talking to on the phone. (And Aunt Mary once again has custody of the fish slippers. Hey, I warned you the analogy was weak.)

Chapter 1. Analogy

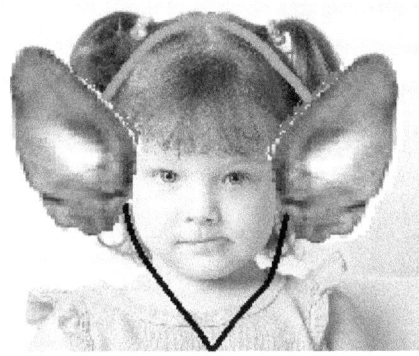

Figure 1-2. Sarah's foam earphones are mounted inside fur-covered giant plastic dog ears that enhance sounds from the direction in which she is looking.

Bone-Conduction Occlusion Effect

Wearing earphones causes bone-conducted sound to increase in loudness, though it's not related to a resonance effect like Sarah's dog earphones. How that works will be covered in Chapters 6 and 9. The phenomenon of sound increasing in loudness when an earphone is in place is called the occlusion effect – the crossed over bone-conduction sound is actually louder in the non-test ear, just as Sarah could hear her mother better than her grandmother can – unless Sarah has the (masking) music on.

Mercifully, this is nearly the end of the analogy, which I hope is some aid in remembering the crossover, crossback, interaural attenuation terminology.

Overview of Masking and Review of Terms

Masking is a difficult topic to fully comprehend. This brief text, and its accompanying games, attempt to make masking easier to understand. We need to mask because sometimes when testing one ear, the signal could **"cross over"** to the non-test ear. We will always put masking in by air-conduction, and preferably using an insert earphone to produce that masking noise. If we aren't using loud enough noise to mask the crossover, then we are **"undermasking."** There are times when the masking noise is so loud it can **"cross back"** to the test ear and cause erroneous results – this is called **overmasking**.

Bone-conduction testing is especially challenging. All of the signal crosses to the non-test ear, and if you insert an earphone to start the masking process, for the low-frequency stimuli, you create a **sound enhancement, called the occlusion effect.** This means you will need even more masking noise in the non-test ear to nullify the occlusion effect. And… unfortunately that added noise makes cross back more likely.

There are **two fundamental approaches to masking: plateau masking and formula masking.** Plateau masking is akin to Sarah's father putting on some music, checking that he can't hear the phone conversation, then turning up the music a bit more to be sure. In plateau masking, you make incremental noise adjustments. In formula masking, you know how your masking is calibrated, and you can calculate how much noise is enough. You'll double check your math – was that really enough (not undermasking), not too much (not overmasking)? This would be like the experienced father knowing that the soundtrack to Nemo (does Nemo have a soundtrack?) at volume 20 will mask the conversation if Sarah's Mom is speaking at 50 dB HL behind a door.

Chapter 1. Analogy

You need to understand plateau masking well before learning about formula masking.

I'll try to make this learning as fun as possible for you – or if that's too high a bar then hopefully this e-book, the games, and the audiometer simulator will make the learning less painful.

Chapter 1. Abbreviations

Abbreviations and Definitions

AC
    air conduction

BC
    bone conduction

Central masking effect
    The elevation of the test ear threshold when masking is heard in the opposite ear, which occurs not because the masking has eliminated the cross hearing, but because the listening task has been made more difficult. It is harder to attend to a very low intensity test signal when hearing noise in the opposite ear, so thresholds increase. Central masking effects are small with low noise levels, and increase as the noise in the non-test ear increases in intensity.

Conservative
    most cautious, careful

Crossback (CB)
    The amount of masking noise that crosses from the non-test ear to the test ear and potentially interferes with hearing of the test ear signal. It is equal to the noise level at the non-test ear minus the air-conduction interaural attenuation.

Crossover (CO)
    The amount of signal that is present in the non-test ear. It is equal to the presentation level of the signal in the test ear minus the interaural attenuation for that transducer.

False Negative Response
    Occurrence of a patient failing to respond to the presentation of a test signal, even though it is above threshold. Occurs due to patient uncertainty, distraction, or presence of increased ambient noise.

False Positive Response
    Occurrence of a patient responding that a tone was heard, when the tone is inaudible. The patient guesses a tone was present when it wasn't. Some patients are more prone to giving false positive responses than other patients.

Interaural Attenuation (IA)
    The amount of sound energy reduction as a signal crosses from the test ear to the non-test ear cochlea (or in the case of overmasking, the noise signal reduction as it crosses from the NTE to the TE cochlea). For pure-tone testing, the minimum interaural attenuation is assumed to be 50 dB for insert earphones, 40 dB for supra-aural earphones and 0 dB when testing via bone-conduction. For speech testing (and speech noise), the minimum insert earphone IA is 60 dB, it is 50 dB for supra-aural earphones.

Chapter 1. Abbreviations

Masking Dilemma

A situation where masking is needed, but using masking causes overmasking. The test needs masking, but using masking will immediately cause overmasking. This is a "no win" situation – I need to mask, I cannot mask. It happens with maximum or near maximum bilateral conductive losses.

Maximum Conductive Loss

A conductive loss of a magnitude that is equal to the interaural attenuation value for the air-conduction transducer being used. (Confusing point: most conductive losses are not more than about 50-60 dB, which is sometimes called a "maximum conductive loss", but for the purposes of a book on masking, we reserve this term for a loss that is so great the stimulus is heard only because the air-conduction signal causes the skull to oscillate, creating a bone-conducted sound that goes to both the test- and non-test ear cochleas.

Non-test ear (NTE)

Ear that is opposite from the one that should be receiving the test stimulus.

Non-test ear air-bone gap (NTE ABG)

The air-conduction threshold minus the bone-conduction threshold for the test ear, which indicates the size of the non-test ear conductive impairment.

Occlusion effect (OE)

Enhancement in the sound received at the cochlea when the external ear is occluded (covered/blocked).

Overmasking (OM)

When the noise presented to the non-test ear crosses back to the test ear, and prevents the hearing of the test ear signal, overmasking is occurring.

Reduced Plateau Width

A normal masking plateau occurs when three consecutive 5-dB increases in masking intensity do not change the hearing threshold. The plateau width is said to be reduced when only one or two 5-dB increases occur before the overmasking portion of the plateau begins.

Sensorineural hearing loss (SNHL)

Hearing loss due to cochlear and/or retrocochlear site of lesion.

Test ear (TE)

Do I really need to define this? Just making sure you can look up the acronym.

Test ear air-bone gap (TE ABG)

The air-conduction threshold minus the bone-conduction threshold for the test ear, which indicates the size of the test ear conductive impairment.

Chapter 1. Abbreviations

Transducer

    In this book, an earphone, headphone or bone oscillator. A transducer converts energy from one form (e.g. electrical) to another form (e.g. acoustic). (Microphones are also transducers.)

Undermasking (UM)

    When the noise presented to the non-test ear is not sufficiently intense to mask the crossed-over signal. If the audiologist undermasks, then the non-test ear is being stimulated; the response does not necessarily reflect the hearing of the test ear.

Chapter 1. Quick Reference

When To Mask – Pure-Tone Testing

When to Mask for Air-Conduction Testing – Summary of Chapter 2

1) If the test ear air-conducted threshold is **50 dB** or more (for insert earphones; or 40 dB or more for supra-aural earphones) above the non-test ear **air**-conduction threshold at the same frequency, then masking is needed.

2) If the test ear air-conduction threshold is **50 dB** or more (for insert earphones; or 40 dB or more for supra-aural earphones) above the non-test ear **bone**-conduction threshold at the same frequency, then masking is needed.

When to Mask for Bone-Conduction Testing – Summary of Chapter 3

1) If there is a 15 dB or more difference between an air-conduction threshold and the unmasked bone-conduction threshold at the same frequency, then use contralateral masking.

Chapter 1. Quick Reference

Plateau Masking Steps

Air-Conduction -- Summary of Chapter 5

- Recognize the need for masking.

- Set the initial masking level at 10 dB above the non-test ear threshold. Re-obtain threshold or check that the threshold has not changed.
- Increase the masking in 5 dB steps, reobtaining the threshold if threshold shifts.
- Continue increasing the masking in 5 dB steps until three consecutive increases in the masking level occurs with no change in hearing threshold.

- If unmasked testing shows bilateral loss, and masked testing shows both ears are 'dead', then it is a masking dilemma

Bone-Conduction - Summary of Chapter 6

- Recognize the need for masking.

- Set the initial masking level at the non-test ear air-conduction threshold, plus 10 dB, plus the occlusion effect size. This book recommends using 20 dB at 250, 10 dB at 500 Hz, and 5 dB at 1000 Hz).

    - If the non-test ear has conductive loss that is larger than the occlusion effect size, you can omit the occlusion effect. The conductive loss will eliminate it.

- Increase the masking in 5 dB steps, re-obtaining threshold if threshold shifts.
- Continue increasing the masking in 5 dB steps until three consecutive increases in the masking level occur with no change in hearing threshold.

- If unmasked testing shows bilateral loss, and masked testing shows both ears are 'dead', then it is a masking dilemma.

Chapter 1. Quick Reference

The Masking Formulae

Pure-Tone Air-Conduction Formula Masking – Summary of Chapter 8

The masking signal must be at or above the minimum, and that minimum level must not be at or above the maximum that protects from overmasking. If the minimum is equal to or greater than maximum, then use plateau masking.

For these formulae, 'TE signal level' is your estimate of the eventual masked threshold.

Minimum Masking Level:
TE signal level – IA + significant NTE ABG + 10 dB

For insert earphones:
TE signal level – 40 dB + NTE ABG

For supra-aural headphones:
TE signal -30 dB + NTE ABG

It is recommended that you use the highest "reasonably possible" AC threshold in this calculation. This way, if your threshold comes in a bit higher than anticipated, you do not need to increase the noise and recheck threshold.

Maximum Masking Level:
BC threshold of the TE + IA – 5

For insert earphones:
BC TE + 45 dB

For supra-aural phones:
BC TE + 35 dB

It is recommended that you use the lowest "reasonably possible" BC threshold – so that if you are wrong, and bone-conduction is a bit better than you assumed, you will not be in an overmasking situation.

Checking Your Masking

Once threshold has been established:

- If the measured threshold comes in <u>better than expected</u>, consider the <u>possibility of overmasking.</u>
  Recheck: BC threshold + 45. If you used masking noise that was louder than this level, you may be overmasking. Lower the masking noise level.

- If threshold is higher <u>than expected (more hearing loss)</u>, consider the <u>possibility of undermasking.</u>
  Recheck: BC threshold – 40 + NTE ABG. If you did not use at least this amount of noise, then increase the masking intensity.

Chapter 1. Quick Reference

Bone-Conduction Formula Masking – Summary of Chapter 9

BC TE is your estimate of the eventual, masked, bone-conduction threshold for the test ear.

Minimum Masking Level:
BC TE +10 + (larger of: OE or NTE ABG)

It is recommended that you use the highest "reasonably possible" BC threshold in this calculation. This way, if your threshold comes in a bit higher than anticipated, you do not need to increase the noise and recheck threshold.

Recommended OE values:
- **250 Hz: 20 dB**
- **500 Hz: 10 dB**
- **1K Hz : 5 dB**
- **2K Hz+: None**

Maximum Masking Level:
BC TE + 45

It is recommended that you use the lowest "reasonably possible" BC threshold – so that if you are wrong, and bone-conduction is a bit better than you assumed, you will not be in an overmasking situation.

Checking Your Masking

Check that masking is sufficient – calculate the Minimum Masking Level using the established BC, and calculate the maximum using that same threshold. The masking level you used must be between Min and Max. If Min > Max then plateau mask, you may have a masking dilemma. (Note, this will only "work" if you use the same threshold for min and max, if you base min and max on different scenarios (e.g. setting min to work in case threshold is a little higher than you guessed, and setting max by thinking about bone-conduction coming in a little better than your best guess) – then this rule does not work.

Chapter 1. Quick Reference

Speech Masking - Summary of Chapter 10

When to Mask

Calculate Signal level – 60 (for insert earphones or 50 for TDH earphones). If that is at or above the NTE BC thresholds for one or more frequency in the 500 to 8k Hz range, then cross hearing may influence your results and masking is warranted.

Masking Formulae

Spondee Threshold

Minimum Masking Level:

Predicted SPONDEE THRESHOLD + 10 dB in case the SPONDEE THRESHOLD is a bit higher than the PTA predicts – IA + largest significant NTE ABG + 10 dB pad

(which gives us)

For insert earphones:
TE estimated SPONDEE THRESHOLD – 40 dB + Largest NTE ABG (500 to 8k Hz)

For supra-aural phones:
TE estimated SPONDEE THRESHOLD – 30 dB + NTE ABG

Word Recognition Testing

Minimum Masking Level:

Presentation level – IA + 10 dB pad

For insert earphones:
TE signal level – 50 dB + Largest NTE ABG (500 to 8k Hz)

For supra-aural phones:
TE signal level – 30 dB + NTE ABG

Maximum Masking Level:

For both spondee threshold and word recognition testing: Best TE BC threshold in the 500-8k Hz range + IA – 5

(which is)

For insert earphones:
Best TE 500-8k Hz + 55 dB

For supra-aural phones:
BC TE + 45 dB

Chapter 1. Quick Reference

Down 20 Rule:

Estimated spondee threshold or word recognition test level – 20 dB.

- Ideal for asymmetrical sensorineural loss.
- If there is test ear conductive loss, this rule can overmask, but the overmasking is usually not consequential – it won't typically interfere with speech understanding.
- Non-test ear conductive loss causes this rule to often give problematic undermasking.

Speech Noise Crossback May Not Alter Results

- Calculate the speech sensation level across frequencies (stimulus level minus TE AC threshold)
- Calculate the theoretical noise crossback level across frequencies (Crossback level minus TE BC threshold)
- So long as the speech is 10 dB more intense than the crossback, test results are unlikely to be influenced by the crossback.

Chapter 2

When Masking is Needed for Air-Conduction Testing

Rules for Future Reference

Compare the test ear air-conduction threshold to

- the non-test ear air-conduction threshold and
- the non-test ear bone-conduction threshold (when available)

If the difference is 50 dB or more (insert earphones, 40 dB for TDH headphones), then masking is needed.

- If the non-test ear immittance is abnormal, then consider need for masking based on the assumption that the non-test ear bone-conduction thresholds are normal.

Interaural Attenuation and Cross-Hearing

Why Masking is Needed

Audiologists put masking noise into the non-test (opposite, contralateral) ear when it is possible that the stimulus is being heard by that non-test ear. When testing by air-conduction, this "cross hearing" occurs when the vibration of the air molecules is intense enough that the skull is set into vibration. The cochlea are embedded within the bones of the skull; once the skull is vibrating, the energy is sent to BOTH the test ear and non-test ear cochleas (Figure 2-1).

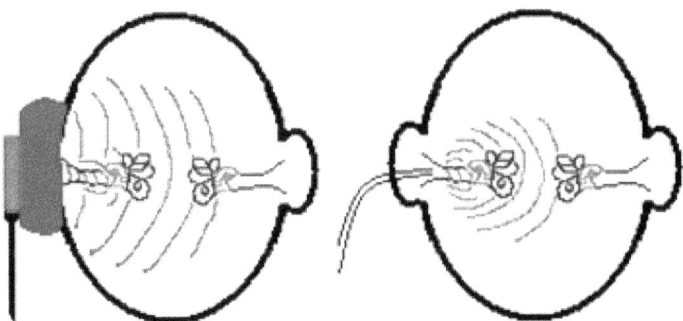

Figure 2-1. The air-conducted test signal, if intense enough, can create vibration of the skull, which permits bone-conduction hearing. Since the skull is fused, this vibration activates fluid motion within both the ipsilateral and the contralateral cochlea: The non-test ear's cochlea is stimulated by bone conduction. Because a sound produced by an insert earphone vibrates only a portion of the ear canal, it takes a greater intensity test signal to create the cross-hearing than if a supra-aural earphone is used.

Chapter 2. When to Mask – Air Conduction

Maximum Conductive Loss

If the sound is loud enough to cross over to the non-test ear, it is also going directly to the test-ear cochlea. When the sound level is above a certain intensity, it will vibrate the skull, and this sound vibration will by-pass the outer and middle ear. This is the concept behind the "maximum conductive loss". A purely conductive loss cannot cause total deafness; the air-conducted sound becomes bone conducted and by-passes the conductive system. (Most conductive loss allows some sound transmission through the middle ear, so the maximum loss usually seen is not a true maximum conductive loss.)

Amount of Crossover

The audiologist's concern is that the bone-conducted sound (created by the loud air-conduction vibration) will be heard by the non-test ear rather than the test ear. If the moderately loud air-conducted sound becomes an above-threshold level bone-conducted sound that is detected by the opposite ear, then the audiologist is not testing the ear to which the stimulus is being sent. In this case, noise needs to be put into the non-test ear to prevent hearing of the crossed-over test ear signal. The amount of noise needed depends on the amount that may be crossing over.

Patients differ in their skin, soft tissue and skull characteristics; not everyone will start to experience cross-hearing at exactly the same intensity level. Studies have been conducted on persons with complete unilateral hearing loss to determine how loud sound has to be in the "dead ear" to be perceived in the good ear. An example audiogram of one such person is shown in Figure 2-2.

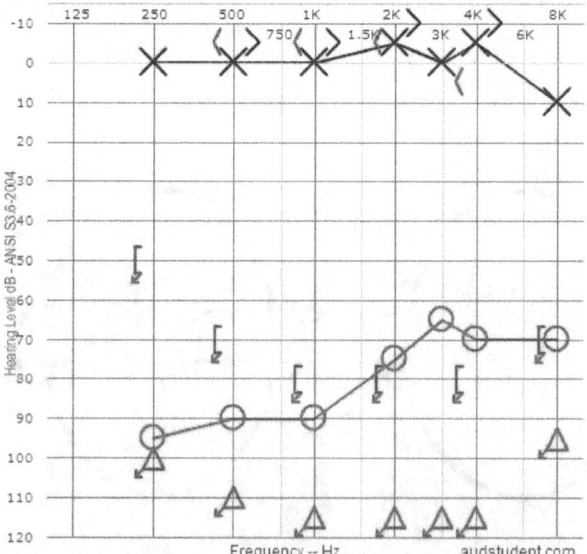

Figure 2-2. Audiogram of a person with unilateral sensorineural hearing loss, shown with and without of the masking of the "dead" right ear. Insert earphones were used.

Defining and Calculating Interaural Attenuation

Recall that the cross hearing for air-conduction occurs when the non-test ear cochlea hears the pure tone sent via the test ear earphone/headphone. The term **interaural attenuation** needs to be defined. It is the **loss** of sound energy that occurs during the process of the sound crossing to the non-test ear cochlea. To determine air-conduction interaural attenuation,

- compare the unmasked air-conduction thresholds of the poorer hearing ear
- to the bone-conduction threshold of the better ear.

In the example above, compare right unmasked air-conduction thresholds to left bone conduction thresholds.

- At 1000 Hz, the right ear unmasked air-conduction threshold is 90,
- the left ear bone-conduction threshold is -5.
- This 95 difference is this patient's interaural attenuation at 1000 Hz.

Interaural attenuation refers to how much sound energy is lost, in this case, as it is transformed from an air-conducted signal to a bone-conducted signal that has crossed the head. When we know the interaural attenuation value, we can determine how loud a sound will be at the non-test ear cochlea (and then, determine if that will be audible or not.) For this patient, if we present a 1000 Hz, 120 dB HL air-conducted pure tone, it will be heard as 25 dB HL (120 – the 95 interaural attenuation) at the non-test cochlea.

Interaural attenuation values vary across patients

Several studies have tested a number of patients with unilateral profound hearing loss to determine the range of interaural attenuation that different patients can have. Figure 2-3A shows the averaged results from some of these studies.

We have no way of knowing before testing a patient if he or she will have low or high interaural attenuation values. You could determine the interaural attenuation if you first test unmasked air conduction and compare the threshold to the better ear's unmasked bone-conduction threshold. (This assumes that after putting masking in the non-test ear the true hearing threshold is even poorer, which means cross hearing did occur.) But that step is not done clinically. It would take too much time and testing.

Since we don't know if the person has a high or low interaural attenuation value before testing, we have to assume the worst-case scenario exists: Assume that the patient you are testing has a low interaural attenuation value – the patient has cross-hearing at the lowest possible level. These levels are shown in Figure 2-3B.

Chapter 2. When to Mask – Air Conduction

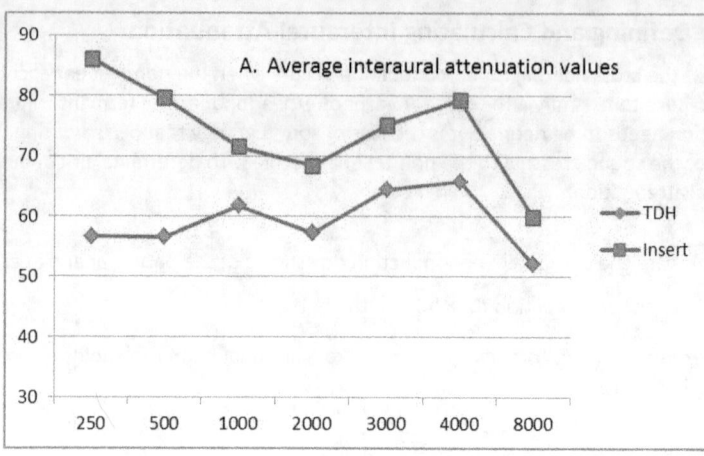

Figure 2-3A. Average interaural attenuation results when testing using supra-aural earphones (a mix of models TDH 39 and 49) and for insert earphones (mix of deeply inserted, shallow insertion, and depth not specified). See reference list for study values used.

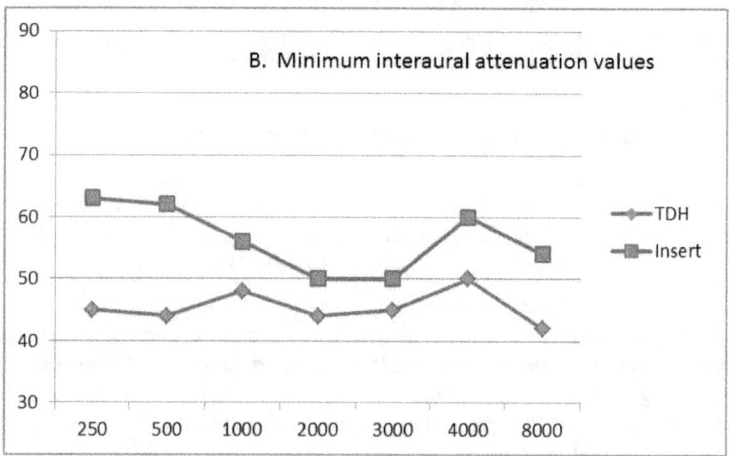

Figure 2-3B. Not everyone has average interaural attenuation values. The lowest values seen in any of the studies is shown.

Chapter 2. When to Mask – Air Conduction

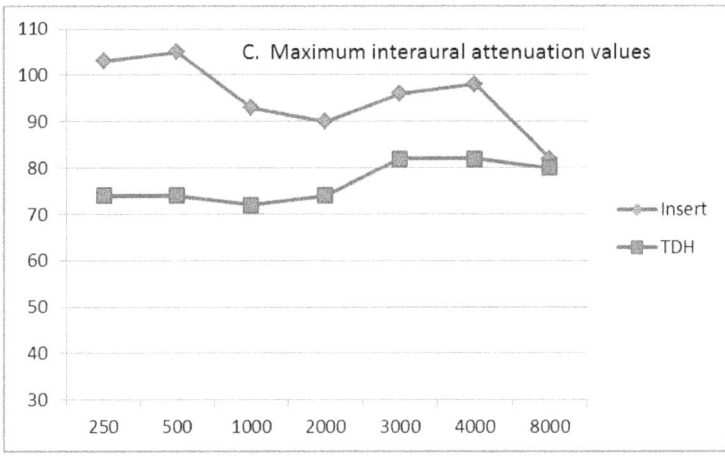

Figure 2-3C. Maximum values (the highest value in any one of the studies) are displayed in this last figure. The total number of subjects tested was 34 for TDH headphones and 40 for insert earphones. See reference list for study values used.

Audiologists have traditionally made the generalization that the lowest interaural attenuation value is 40 dB for supra-aural earphones and 50 dB for insert earphones. These assumptions are very cautious (conservative). In the vast majority of cases, the value will be higher. Figure 2-3C shows that for some patients, interaural attenuation values for insert earphones can exceed 100 dB.

Although interaural attenuation varies with frequency, most audiologists ignore this fact

In reviewing Figure 2-3B, you see that the minimum interaural attenuation for insert earphones is 50 dB only for 2000 and 3000 Hz. One could use the chart below of the minimum interaural attenuation values per frequency, and only use contralateral masking if the signal level is high enough that there may be cross hearing at that frequency. However, in the professional communities in which I have worked, this is not typically done. Therefore, if I were to use this (scientifically sound) technique, my colleagues might question what I was doing, and a few might question my competence. Since masking is really not that hard (trust me, it soon won't be), it's not all that onerous to assume that the interaural attenuation could be as low as 50 dB for insert earphones and use this value when masking, regardless of frequency. However, there will be times when you may want to know what those minimum levels really are; the next section summarizes them to serve as an easy reference.

Chapter 2. When to Mask – Air Conduction

Frequency-Specific Minimal IA Values

Table 2-1. Minimal frequency-specific IA value summary (rounded values, in dB).

Frequency (Hz)	250	500	1k	2k	3k	4k	8k
Inserts	60	60	55	50	50	60	55
TDH	45	45	45	45	45	50	40

The Practical Part: Determining When Air-Conducted Masking is Needed

If the Test Ear Air-Conduction Threshold is at Least 50 dB More Than the Opposite Ear's Air-Conduction Threshold or Bone-Conduction Threshold, Then Masking is Needed.

The general rule is to compare the air-conduction threshold of the test ear to air-conduction threshold of the non-test ear. If the test ear threshold is ≥ 50 dB above the non-test ear threshold, then masking is needed. However, if the non-test ear has conductive hearing loss, and thus better bone-conduction sensitivity than air-conduction sensitivity, then the "compare air to air" rule will not detect all the times when masking is needed. Observe Figure 2-4.

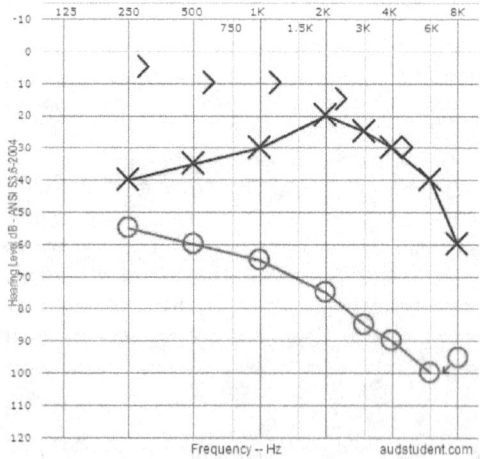

Figure 2-4. Using the "mask the non-test ear when testing the poorer ear if the air-conduction thresholds differ by 50 dB or more" rule would not alert the audiologist that the low-frequency thresholds of the right ear may also be due to potential for cross-hearing. The secondary rule is to "mask the non-test ear when testing the poorer ear if the air-conduction threshold is 50 dB or more higher than the **bone**-conduction threshold of the non-test ear."

Chapter 2. When to Mask – Air Conduction

Using Immittance Testing to Predict When Masking Will Be Needed

Since air-conduction testing is conducted (in most clinics) before bone-conduction testing, it's hard to know when the "mask if the air-conduction thresholds are 50 or more dB above the non-test ear bone-conduction threshold" rule is going to be applied. If immittance test results are available, they can be used to alert you that bone-conduction thresholds may be better than the air-conduction thresholds. For example, if the left ear had an abnormal tympanogram, and absent left ipsilateral reflexes, then the alert audiologist would consider the possibility of left conductive loss, and make the preliminary conclusion that bone-conduction results may be normal. The audiologist assumes the bone-conduction thresholds will be 0 dB HL (or perhaps even better, if the patient is a child). The audiologist then determines whether the other ear's air-conduction threshold is 50 dB or higher. If so, then the test ear signal may be crossing over, and based on these preliminary results, it would be assumed that contralateral masking is needed. (To restate, using the above example where the left ear's loss is presumed to be conductive, when testing the right ear by air-conduction, as soon as a right ear threshold is measured at 50 dB HL or higher, the audiologist would mask the left ear when testing the right ear.) There is no harm in masking when not needed, other than it takes additional time.

Review Complete Test Results to Ensure Air-Conduction Masking Was Conducted as Needed

It's prudent to review the completed audiogram before ending testing, to double check that masking was conducted when needed. Once all the bone-conduction thresholds have been obtained, it is easy to see if you have forgotten to mask based on the "test-ear air to non-test ear bone" rule.

Assume Unmasked Bone-Conduction Thresholds Are the Non-Test Ear's Thresholds When Determining Need for Masking

Note that in Figure 2-4 unmasked bone-conduction scores are shown. How do you know if that's really the left cochlea's hearing sensitivity? You don't. But since it **could** be the left ear, then we need to mask.

Second "When to Mask for AC" Reiterated

For clarity then, let's state the second "when to mask for air-conduction" rule again. If there is a 50 dB or more difference between an air-conduction test ear threshold and the non-test ear bone-conduction threshold, then masking is needed. And if there may be this size difference, it's prudent to mask rather than waiting until all the bone-conduction thresholds are obtained.

Need Some Practice? There's an App / Game for That

How to Use the Masking Calculator

The Masking Calculator (mCalc) is an app that allows you to check whether masking is needed. This would be a good time to start using the app. Note that you adjust the air- and bone-conduction thresholds: The masked/unmasked symbols are not used. In this application, you are doing a "what if" and assuming that the thresholds are as they would be if masking were used – the levels you adjust in the app are assumed to be the "real"

Chapter 2. When to Mask – Air Conduction

thresholds. You can input impossible scenarios, such as a unilateral profound conductive loss, if you desire.

The masking calculator is at this Web location: http://www.audsim.com/mcalc/mCalc.html

At this stage of learning, you should adjust the thresholds and click on the "Mask Air" buttons. As shown in Figure 2-5, the interaural attenuation is always assumed to be 50 dB for air-conduction. The crossover will be calculated and displayed next to the non-test ear bone conduction threshold (shown as "Co" in the app). If the crossover is above the bone-conduction threshold, masking is recommended.

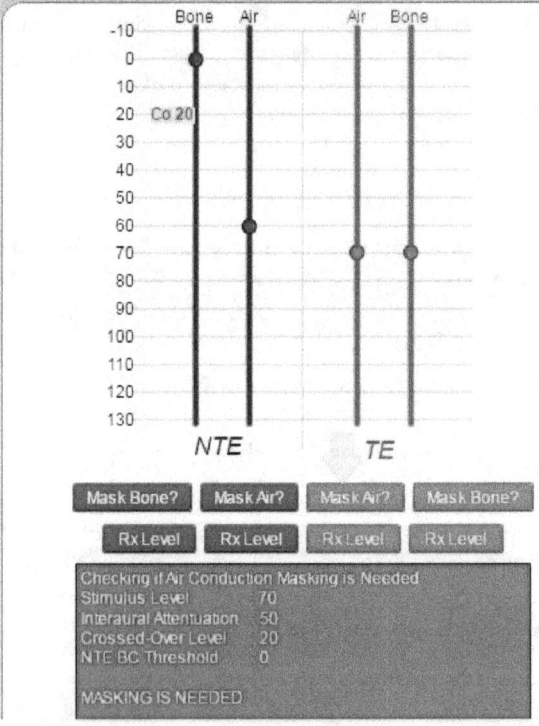

Figure 2-5. Screen shot of the mCalc application. Click on "Mask Air?" to determine if masking is needed. If the air-conduction threshold of the poorer ear is 50 dB or more above the bone-conduction threshold of the better ear, then masking is needed. Use this app to examine different scenarios to see if you correctly predict when masking is and is not needed.

mQuest Game

There is a game that tests you on the mCalc concepts. Level 1 of the Game-Based Learning App, called mQuest, gives you practice at recognizing when to mask in cases of sensorineural loss: the first "when to mask rule" is sufficient (50 dB or more difference between air-conduction thresholds). Levels 2 and 3 may require use of the second rule (compare test ear air to non-test ear bone); the examples include mixed loss. Note that air-bone gaps in the test ear are irrelevant. You will compare the **air**-conduction threshold of the **test** ear (whether or not it has a conductive component) to the **bone**-conduction threshold of the **non-test** ear. 100% mastery is needed to move up in game levels.

Chapter 2. When to Mask – Air Conduction

A Review of the Key Points

- Air-conduction cross over (cross hearing) occurs when the skull vibrates, so the signal is crossing over by bone conduction.

- Compare the air-conduction test ear threshold to the bone-conduction threshold of the opposite ear. If there is a 50 dB difference, masking is needed.
- If there is reason to suspect that the non-test ear has conductive loss, assume that bone-conduction thresholds are normal. Test with contralateral masking if your air-conduction thresholds are 50 dB or higher.
- Once you obtain the better ear's unmasked bone-conduction threshold, determine if any of the poorer ear's air-conduction thresholds are 50 dB or more higher than those bone-conduction thresholds. If so, then masking is needed.
- When to Mask:
    - If the test ear air-conducted threshold is **50 dB** or more (for insert earphones; or 40 dB or more for supra-aural earphones) above the non-test ear **air**-conduction threshold at the same frequency, then masking is needed
    - If the test ear air-conduction threshold is **50**dB or more (for insert earphones; or 40 dB or more for supra-aural earphones) above the non-test ear **bone**-conduction threshold at the same frequency, then masking is needed.

References:

The data for Figure 2-3 are derived from these articles.

Brannstrom, K.J. & Lantz, J. (2010) Interaural attenuation for Sennheiser HAD 200 circumaural earphones. *International Journal of Audiology, 49,* 467-471.

Munro, K.J. & Agnew, N. (1999). A comparison of the interaural attenuation with the Etymotic ER-3A insert earphone and the Telephonics TDH-39 supra-aural earphone. *British Journal of Audiology, 33*(4), 259-262.

Munro, K.J., & Contractor, A. (2010). Inter-aural attenuation with insert earphones. *International Journal of Audiology, 49,* 799-801.

Sklare, D.A., & Denenberg, L.J. (1987). Interaural attenuation for tubephone insert earphones. *Ear and Hearing, 8*(5), 298-300.

Chapter 3

When to Mask for Bone-Conduction Testing

When to Mask Rule

If there is a 15 dB or more difference between the test-ear air-conduction threshold and the unmasked bone-conduction threshold at the same frequency, then test-ear bone-conduction masking is needed.

Bone-Conduction Interaural Attenuation is Assumed to be 0 dB HL

Because the bones of the adult head are fused at the cranial sutures, it's generally stated that if you vibrate one bone of the head, you will vibrate them all equally. This means that if you put the bone oscillator on the right mastoid, the vibration goes to both cochleas. Therefore, there is no interaural attenuation in bone-conduction testing. That statement is not completely true. There can be some interaural attenuation for bone conduction, but it's typically not a lot – usually 10 dB or less. Examine Figure 3-1, the same audiogram shown in the prior chapter, and note that 4000 Hz shows 15 dB of interaural attenuation for bone conduction.

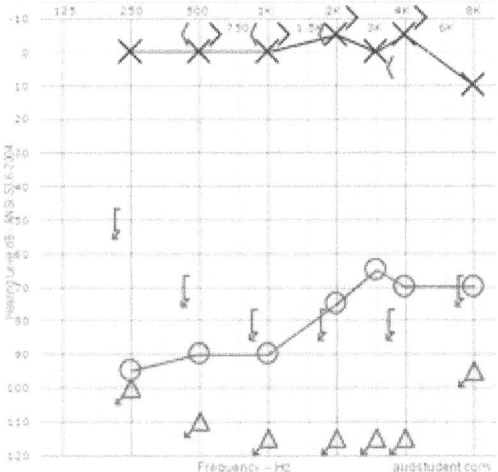

Figure 3-1. At 4000 Hz the right ear unmasked bone-conduction threshold is 5 dB, which is 15 dB higher than the left ear unmasked threshold. This shows that this patient has 15 dB of interaural attenuation. However, at the other frequencies, the interaural attenuation is 0 dB HL. The most conservative (careful) approach is to assume there is no interaural attenuation – that the entire intensity of the sound is carried to the non-test ear.

When to Mask Bone Conduction – Some Advocate "Always"

The 2004 American National Standards Institute (ANSI) audiometric calibration standards assume that masking was used when testing bone-conduction hearing. Introducing masking noise to the non-test ear makes the listening task a little harder for a patient – it elevates the test ear threshold slightly relative to the threshold that would be obtained without putting noise in the opposite ear. This is called the **central masking effect**. It's a small effect when the contralateral noise is at near-threshold-levels, but it often creates a 5 dB elevation of threshold. The fact that ANSI assumes you are always using contralateral masking means that if you don't test using contralateral masking, bone-conduction thresholds may well be 5 dB better. (The threshold will not be elevated by the central masking effect.) The person with perfectly normal hearing would have thresholds of -5 dB HL, not 0 dB HL. (Note again, Figure 3-1.) This can create the appearance of minor air-bone gaps. This is one reason that some audiologists advocate masking bone-conduction thresholds routinely.

Another argument for using masking, and for testing bone conduction in each ear, is the definition of a complete hearing test: air- and bone-conduction threshold testing in each ear. If taken literally, this would require testing each ear's bone-conduction thresholds, using contralateral masking to ensure that one is indeed testing the ear that one intends to test. However, that means conducting more testing than needed, which is an inconvenience to both the patient and audiologist.

When Is Masking Necessary? To Document an Air-Bone Gap in the Test Ear

When testing bone-conduction hearing without masking, the sound is of similar intensity at each cochlea since interaural attenuation is ~0 dB. If there is a better hearing ear, then that is the cochlea that detects the signal. I'm assuming you know the definition of conductive involvement: an air-bone gap of 15 dB or more. (If not, you're not ready to study masking.) If the unmasked bone-conduction test results rule out conductive involvement, then no further testing is needed. If there is a possibility of conductive loss, then we need to know whether the air-bone gaps are unilateral or bilateral.

Examine Figure 3-2. The loss is bilateral and symmetrical. No information would be gained by testing the left ear by bone-conduction. It cannot be significantly better than the unmasked right ear thresholds, since bone-conduction interaural attenuation is usually 0 dB and seldom more than 10 dB. Bone-conduction masking is not needed.

Chapter 3. When to Mask – Bone Conduction

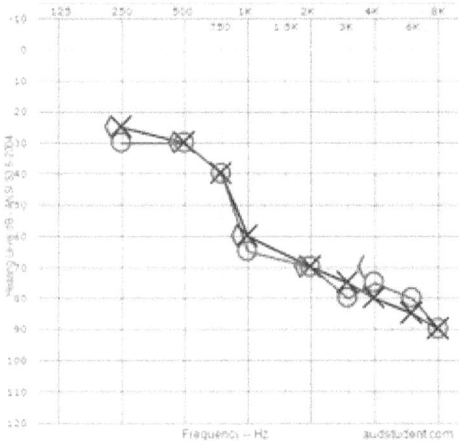

Figure 3-2. There is no need to mask the right ear bone-conduction thresholds, or to test the left ear bone-conduction thresholds. Since the unmasked bone-conduction thresholds represent the better cochlea if there is one, the left ear's bone conduction thresholds will not show a conductive component even if it were to be tested.

In contrast, Figure 3-3 shows a case where bone-conduction masking is needed. There may be air-bone gaps for both the right and left ears.

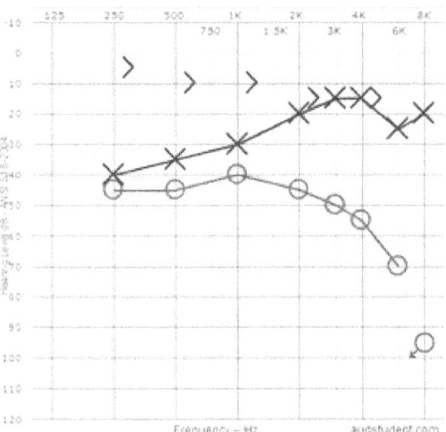

Figure 3-3. Masking is needed for bone-conduction testing for each ear. In the left ear, there are apparent air-bone gaps at 1000 Hz and below, but the bone-conduction thresholds may reflect the right ear's cochlear sensitivity. Left ear bone-conduction testing requires that masking noise be put into the right ear to prevent it from detecting the crossed-over bone conduction signal, in case the right ear cochlea does have normal hearing. The right ear also requires masked bone-conduction testing at all frequencies. If the bone oscillator were placed on the right mastoid, similar or identical unmasked thresholds would be obtained, and again, it would not be known if the thresholds were truly for the right cochlea, or if it was a cross-hearing response from the left cochlea.

Chapter 3. When to Mask – Bone Conduction

Formal Statement of the "When Is Masking Needed for Bone-Conduction" Rule

- If there is (or if there is a potential for) a 15 dB or more air-bone gap, mask.
- Specifically, if there is a 15 dB or more difference between an air-conduction threshold and the unmasked bone-conduction threshold, then use contralateral masking.

The rule for when to mask is "if you need to determine if there is truly a conductive hearing loss, if you aren't sure which cochlea is responding and it matters, then mask." We can make the rule even more specific – mask if there is any possibility there could be a 15 dB or more air-bone gap. Because it is traditional to start testing bone-conduction without masking, the findings as shown in Figure 3-3 are typical. We don't yet know if there is or is not an air-bone gap without having yet masked, so we can also say <u>if there is a 15 dB or more difference between an air-conduction threshold and the unmasked bone-conduction threshold, then use contralateral masking.</u>

Using mCalc and the mQuest Game-Based Learning System

The mCalc app can again be used to allow you to experiment with different air- and bone-conduction thresholds to see if you can recognize when masking is needed. As noted in the last chapter, the app notes the "air" and "bone" thresholds. Note that it doesn't give masked and unmasked symbols. mQuest shows an audiogram, but only one frequency. In these respects, the app and game are different from what you will experience in clinical testing. You'll also need to practice recognizing when masking is needed when viewing in the traditional audiogram format, which is done in the next chapter.

It is recommended that you begin recognizing when to mask by using the app and playing the mQuest game, levels 4 and 5. Once you have reached proficiency with the app and games, go on to Chapter 4.

Chapter 3. When to Mask – Bone Conduction

Key Concepts

- The adult skull is fused, so if you place the bone vibrator on one mastoid, the bone-conducted signal goes to both mastoids and thus, stimulates both cochlea.

- The unmasked bone-conduction threshold indicates the better ear's hearing (if there is one ear that is better than the other).
- If the loss is sensorineural and bilaterally symmetrical or if hearing is normal bilaterally, then masking for bone-conduction testing is not needed: you have already ruled out conductive involvement. There is no possibility of air-bone gaps.
- When there is an apparent air-bone gap between an unmasked bone-conduction threshold and the air-conduction threshold of the test ear, use masking in the contralateral ear so that you can ensure that you are finding the test ear's threshold.

- The masking rule is:

  If there is a 15 dB or more difference between an air-conduction threshold and the unmasked bone-conduction threshold at the same frequency, then use contralateral masking.

32

Chapter 4

Recognizing the Need for Masking

Overview

Because the mCalc app does not use standard audiometric symbols, and the mQuest game shows only one frequency of the audiogram, this chapter reviews 'when to mask' using the traditional audiogram. Both air- and bone-conduction need for masking are tested. Assume insert earphones were used. The masking rules to use are as follows:

1. For air-conduction, if the poorer ear threshold is 50 or more dB worse than the better ear AIR-conduction threshold, then masking is needed in the non-test ear.
2. For air-conduction, if the poorer ear threshold is 50 or more dB worse than the better ear BONE-conduction threshold, then masking is needed in the non-test ear.
3. For bone-conduction testing, if there is, or if there is the possibility of, a 15 dB or greater air-bone gap in the test ear, then the non-test ear needs to be masked.

Assume Use of Insert Earphones

Question 1

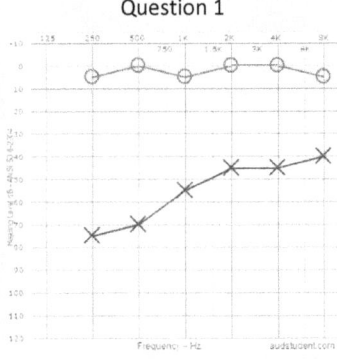

Figure 4-1. At which frequencies is masking required for air-conduction testing?

Click all that apply

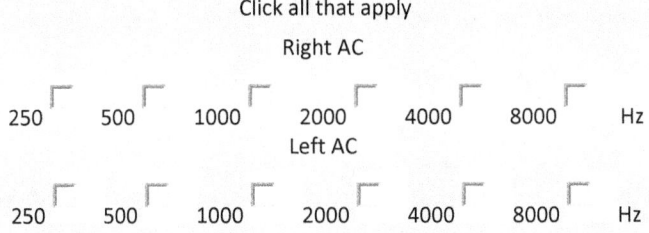

Which ear would receive the masking noise, and would that be input by air- or bone-conduction?

Chapter 4. Practice – Recognizing Need for Masking

Answer 4-1

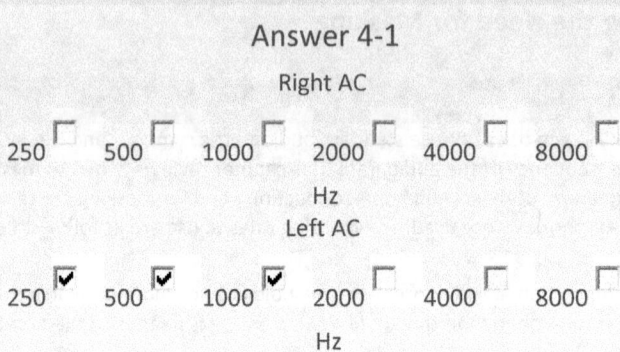

Use rule 1: For air-conduction, if the poorer ear threshold is 50 or more dB worse than the better ear AIR-conduction threshold, then masking is needed in the non-test ear.

The masking would be put into the RIGHT ear, by AIR-conduction.

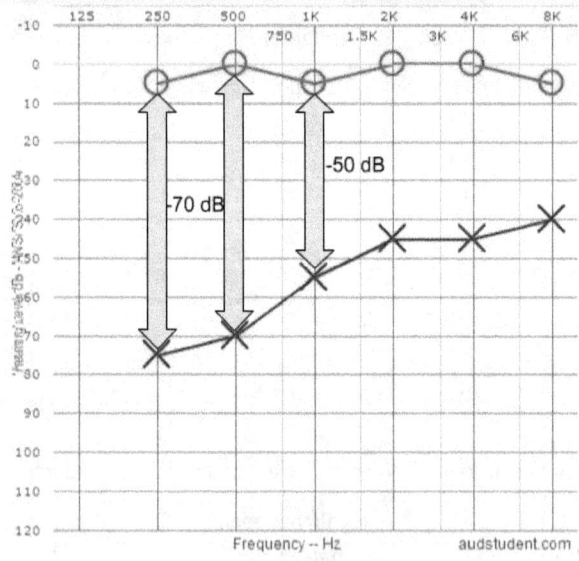

Chapter 4. Practice – Recognizing Need for Masking

Question 2

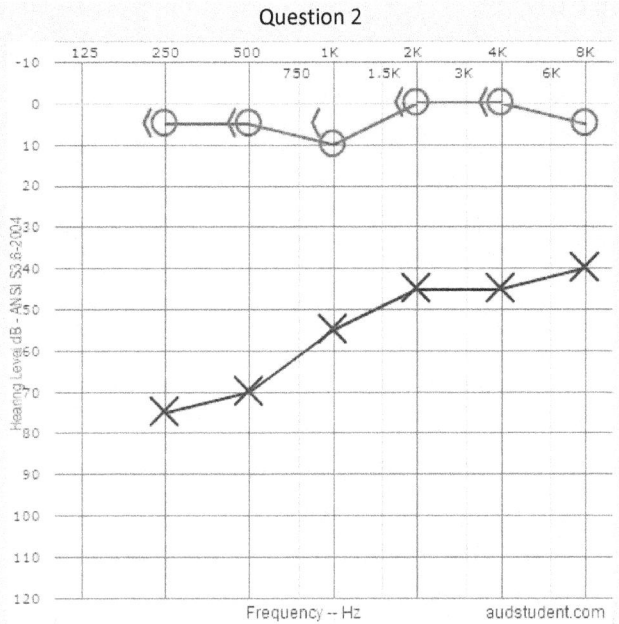

Figure 4-2. At which frequencies is masking required for air-conduction testing?

Click all that apply

Right AC

☐ 250 ☐ 500 ☐ 1000 ☐ 2000 ☐ 4000 ☐ 8000 Hz

Left AC

☐ 250 ☐ 500 ☐ 1000 ☐ 2000 ☐ 4000 ☐ 8000 Hz

Which ear would receive the masking noise, and would that be input by air- or bone-conduction?

Chapter 4. Practice – Recognizing Need for Masking

Answer 4-2

Right AC

☐ 250   ☐ 500   ☐ 1000   ☐ 2000   ☐ 4000   ☐ 8000   Hz

Left AC

☑ 250   ☑ 500   ☑ 1000   ☐ 2000   ☐ 4000   ☐ 8000   Hz

Use rule 2: For air-conduction, if the poorer ear threshold is 50 or more dB worse than the better ear BONE-conduction threshold, then masking is needed in the non-test ear. Note that rule 1 (compare air to air) would not have shown the need for masking at 1000 Hz.

The masking would be put into the RIGHT ear, by AIR-conduction.

Question 3

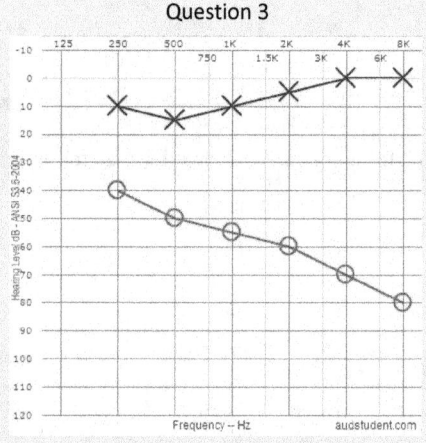

Figure 4-3

At which frequencies is masking required for air-conduction testing?

Click all that apply

Right AC

☐ 250   ☐ 500   ☐ 1000   ☐ 2000   ☐ 4000   ☐ 8000

Hz

Left AC

☐ 250   ☐ 500   ☐ 1000   ☐ 2000   ☐ 4000   ☐ 8000

Hz

Chapter 4. Practice – Recognizing Need for Masking

Which ear would receive the masking noise, and would that be input by air- or bone-conduction?

Answer 4-3

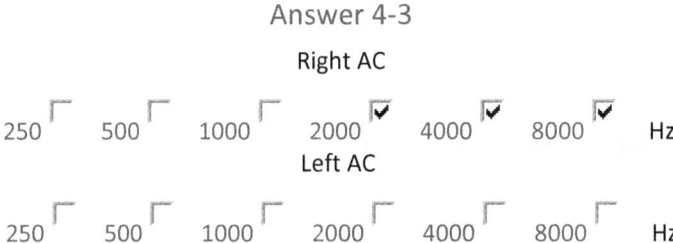

Use rule 1: For air-conduction, if the poorer ear threshold is 50 or more dB worse than the better ear AIR-conduction threshold, then masking is needed in the non-test ear.

The masking would be put into the LEFT ear, by AIR-conduction.

Question 4

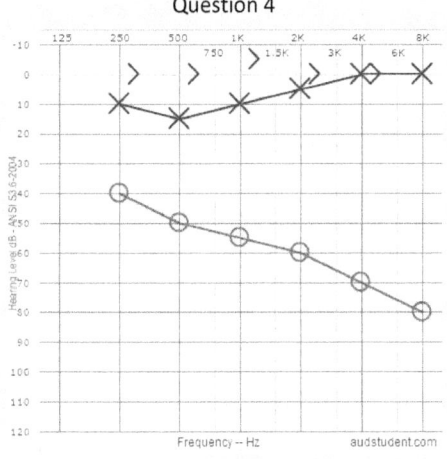

Figure 4-4

At which frequencies is masking required for air-conduction testing?

Click all that apply

Right AC

☐ 250   ☐ 500   ☐ 1000   ☐ 2000   ☐ 4000   ☐ 8000   Hz

Left AC

☐ 250   ☐ 500   ☐ 1000   ☐ 2000   ☐ 4000   ☐ 8000   Hz

Chapter 4. Practice – Recognizing Need for Masking

Which ear would receive the masking noise, and would that be input by air- or bone-conduction?

Answer 4-4

Right AC

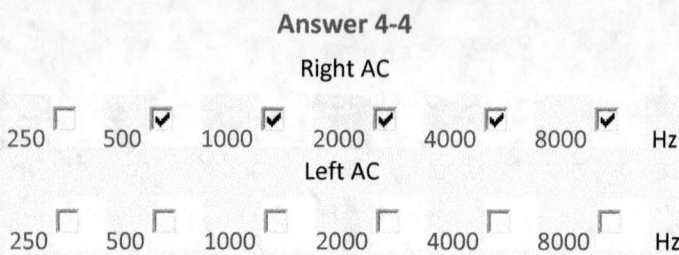

250 ☐ 500 ☑ 1000 ☑ 2000 ☑ 4000 ☑ 8000 ☑ Hz

Left AC

250 ☐ 500 ☐ 1000 ☐ 2000 ☐ 4000 ☐ 8000 ☐ Hz

Use rule 2. For air-conduction, if the poorer ear threshold is 50 or more dB worse than the better ear BONE-conduction threshold, then masking is needed in the non-test ear. Note that rule 1 (compare air to air) would not have shown the need for masking at 500 and 1000 Hz.

The masking would be put into the LEFT ear, by AIR-conduction.

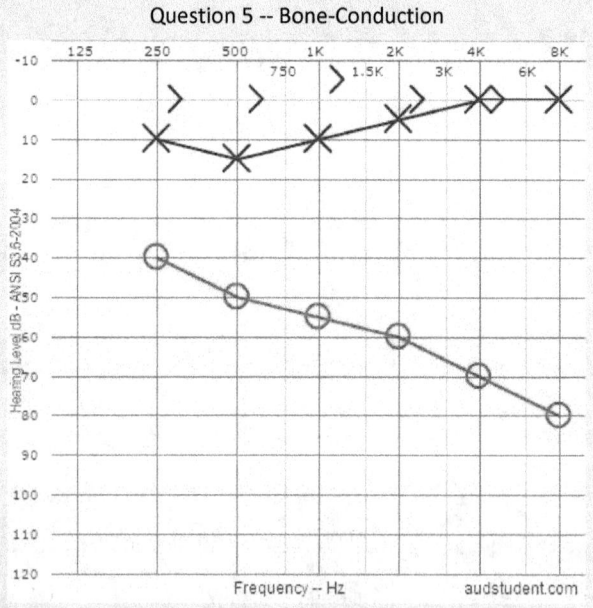

Figure 4-5

For this next example, we switch to bone-conduction masking. At which frequencies is masking required for bone-conduction testing?

Right BC

Chapter 4. Practice – Recognizing Need for Masking

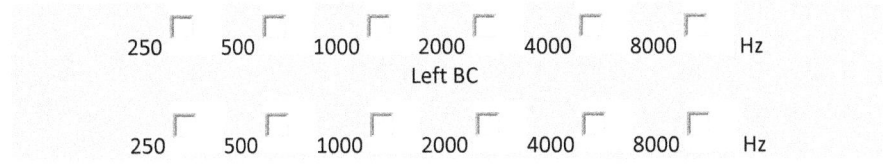

Answer 4-5

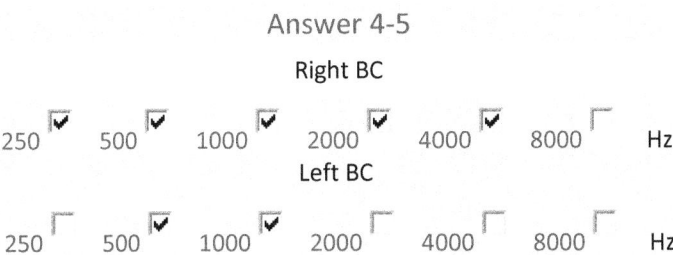

Use rule 3: For bone-conduction testing, if there is, or if there is the possibility of, a 15 dB or greater air-bone gap in the test ear, then the non-test ear needs to be masked.

The left ear shows an air-bone gap between the unmasked left ear bone-conduction threshold and the left air-conduction threshold at 500 and 1000 Hz. Since the bone-conduction testing is unmasked, the results could be for the right ear, and therefore there is need to mask the contralateral ear when conducting the bone-conduction testing on the right ear.

8 kHz is not traditionally tested by bone-conduction.

When masking is needed for the left ear bone-conduction threshold testing, the masking is put into the right ear by AIR conduction.

When masking is needed for the right bone-conduction threshold testing, the masking is put into the left ear by AIR conduction

Chapter 4. Practice – Recognizing Need for Masking

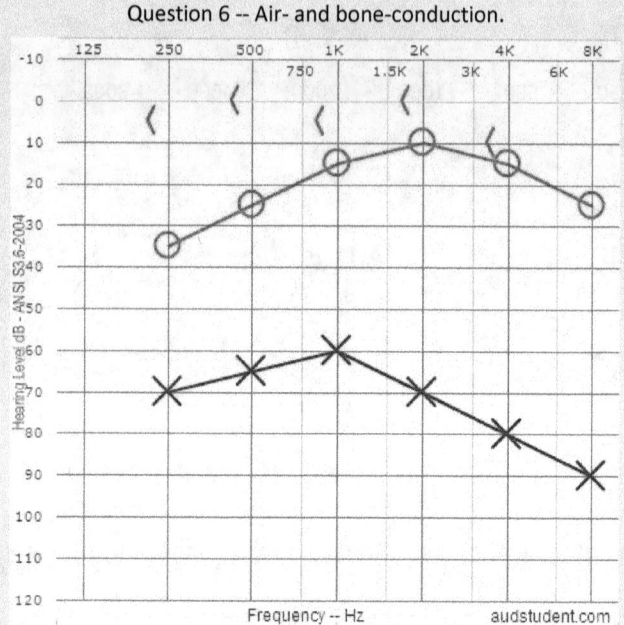

Figure 4-6

At which frequencies is masking required for air- and bone-conduction testing?

Click all that apply

Right AC

250 ☐ 500 ☐ 1000 ☐ 2000 ☐ 4000 ☐ 8000 ☐ Hz

Left AC

250 ☐ 500 ☐ 1000 ☐ 2000 ☐ 4000 ☐ 8000 ☐ Hz

Right BC

250 ☐ 500 ☐ 1000 ☐ 2000 ☐ 4000 ☐ 8000 ☐ Hz

Left BC

250 ☐ 500 ☐ 1000 ☐ 2000 ☐ 4000 ☐ 8000 ☐ Hz

Answer 4-6

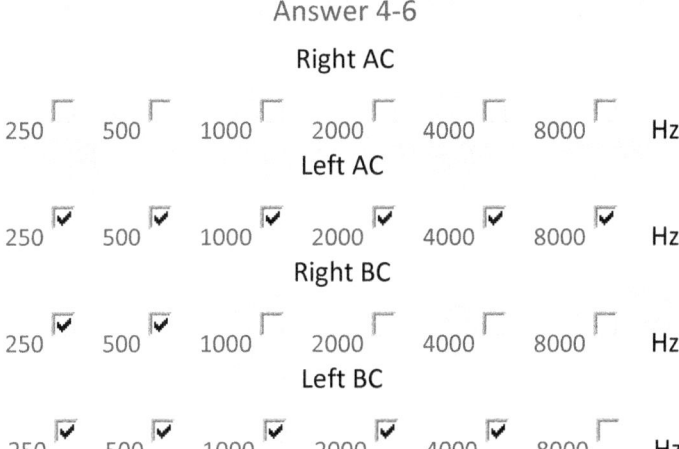

Notes: right bone conduction testing at 1k and 2k shows only a 10 dB air-bone gap; the gap must be significant – 15 dB or greater – in order for masking to be required. The second masking rule alerts you to the need for masking at 1000 Hz for left air-conduction testing; the two air-conduction thresholds only differ by 45 dB, but the left air to unmasked bone-conduction threshold difference is 55 dB.

Chapter 4. Practice – Recognizing Need for Masking

Question 7 -- Determining Need for 8kHz Air-Conduction Masking.

This next case is a special case – as you examine what needs masking, carefully consider if you need to mask when testing 8k Hz by air-conduction. (Bone-conduction testing is usually not conducted at 8k Hz.)

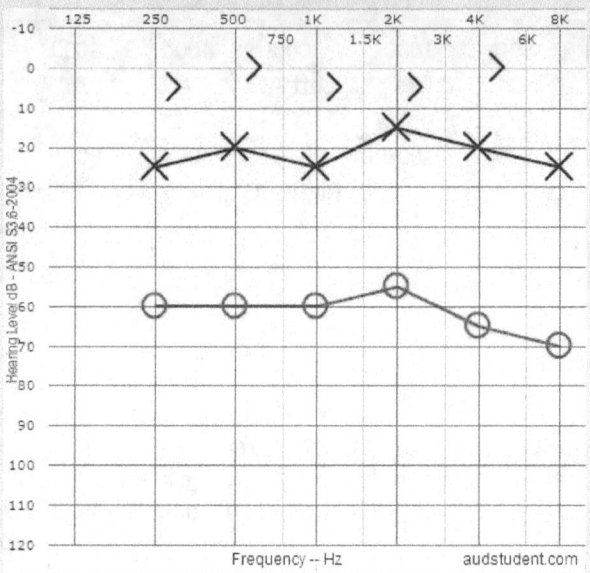

Figure 4-7

At which frequencies is masking required for air- and bone-conduction testing?

Click all that apply

Right AC

☐ 250   ☐ 500   ☐ 1000   ☐ 2000   ☐ 4000   ☐ 8000   Hz

Left AC

☐ 250   ☐ 500   ☐ 1000   ☐ 2000   ☐ 4000   ☐ 8000   Hz

Right BC

☐ 250   ☐ 500   ☐ 1000   ☐ 2000   ☐ 4000   ☐ 8000   Hz

Left BC

☐ 250   ☐ 500   ☐ 1000   ☐ 2000   ☐ 4000   ☐ 8000   Hz

Chapter 4. Practice – Recognizing Need for Masking

Answer 4-7

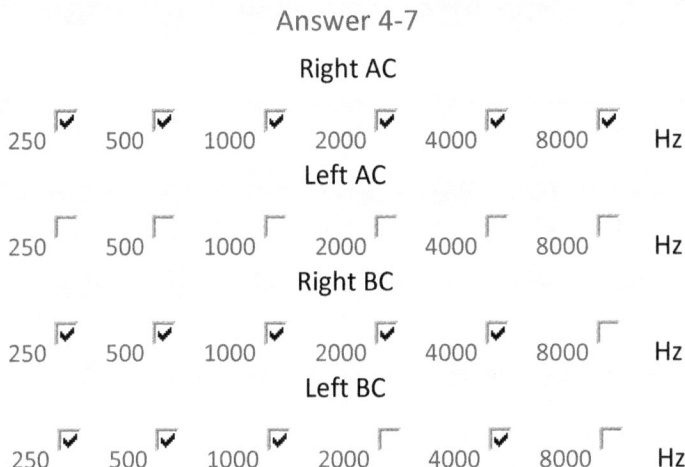

Note that masking rule 2 asks you to compare the air-conduction threshold to the bone-conduction threshold, but you cannot test bone-conduction hearing at 8000 Hz. (Actually, many audiometers allow this testing now, but audiologists do not test 8000 Hz bone conduction routinely.) Bone-conduction testing measures cochlear sensitivity; regardless of whether we test 8k Hz, the cochlea hears by bone-conduction at this frequency. Mentally project the "bone line" out to 8000 Hz – use your guess of the 8000 Hz bone-conduction threshold to determine if masking should be used.

Because bone-conduction is not traditionally tested at 8000 Hz, the table above does not list bone-conduction masking as needed for this frequency.

Chapter 4. Practice – Recognizing Need for Masking

Key Points

- Use the three masking rules in determining need for masking.

- Masking is always input by air-conduction, to the non-test ear; this is true regardless of whether testing air- or bone-conduction hearing.

- Bone-conduction hearing is not routinely tested at 8000 Hz, but consider the bone-conduction threshold that would probably be found when examining need for air-conduction threshold testing masking. If the "air to bone" difference would be 50 dB or greater if bone-conduction had been tested at 8000 Hz, then masking for air-conduction is appropriate.

Chapter 5

Plateau Masking for Air-Conduction Testing

Quick Reference – AC Plateau Masking Steps

- Recognize the need for masking.
- Set the initial masking level at 10 dB above the non-test ear threshold.
- Re-obtain threshold.
- Increase the masking in 5 dB steps, obtaining threshold each time (or ensuring that the threshold did not change.)
- Continue increasing the masking in 5 dB steps until three consecutive increases in the masking level occurs with no change in hearing threshold.

Conductive loss, both when in the test ear and when in the non-test ear, narrows the masking plateau. Bilateral conductive loss may create a masking dilemma where you initially find bilateral conductive loss and after masking have two "dead" ears. There is no solution to a true masking dilemma where the loss size is equal to the interaural attenuation. You can increase interaural attenuation by inserting the insert earphones as deeply as possible.

Overview

Plateau masking, or the Hood plateau method, is the time honored, gold-standard of masking approaches. Masking is put into the non-test ear and gradually increased while determining if there is a shift in the test ear threshold. The procedures are fairly straight-forward. This chapter will discuss the procedure and overview use of the audstudent.com audiometer simulator, which can be used to practice plateau masking.

Before the plateau approach can be understood, there are a few fundamentals to cover.

Definition of "dB Effective Masking Level" (dB EM)

While thresholds are measured in dB HL, the masking level intensity calibration is dB EM, which stands for "effective masking," an unfortunate name choice in my opinion. If you say "I used X dB effective masking" you might think it means you were effectively preventing cross hearing, but dB EM is just an intensity standard, and it does not imply that you are correctly/effectively masking.

Even if the name is not ideal, the way the audiometer is calibrated is convenient. A 20 dB EM masking noise will mask a 20 dB HL tone, if the two sounds are put into the same ear. For example, route a 20 dB HL pure tone to your right ear, and set the left channel of the audiometer to 20 dB EM and then route that to the right ear instead of the left ear. If you are correctly calibrated, you hear the noise, but are not be able to detect the tone. (If you

Chapter 5. Air-Conduction Plateau Masking

increase the tone to 25 dB HL, it becomes audible.) That is a way to check that your audiometer's calibration, but of course it is not the way you use masking: the noise is routed to the contralateral ear

Why dB EM is Used

When masking is needed, we are concerned about the test ear signal having crossed to the non-test ear cochlea. If you have crossover to the non-test ear cochlea that is 20 dB HL, that sound will be masked with 20 dB EM that reaches the non-test ear cochlea. And of course, this holds at all intensities: if you have 40 dB HL of crossover to the non-test ear (NTE) cochlea, then it will be rendered inaudible by 40 dB EM noise at that same cochlea. In the formula masking section of this e-book, we'll use this concept to our benefit. If we can calculate how much crossover is at the non-test ear cochlea, then we can figure out how much noise to put into the non-test ear to ensure the crossover is masked. However, before formula masking can be mastered, it helps to fully understand plateau masking.

They key point at this moment is that dB EM is just an intensity level, and "effective" doesn't necessarily mean you have effectively masked.

Central Masking

Central masking is an increase in the test ear threshold that occurs when noise is put into the opposite ear -- just because the listening task has been made harder.

The brain receives input from both ears, having masking noise in the opposite ear makes it harder to detect near-threshold level sounds in the test ear.

When you put masking into the non-test ear, you may see an initial 5 dB threshold increase that is just due to the increased difficulty of "signal detection" task. That minor increase in threshold is not proof that the signal was crossing over without masking.

Central masking can increase the non-test ear threshold or the test ear threshold. The signal will need to be louder to be heard – regardless of whether it is detected in the test ear or in the non-test ear.

Undermasking Underestimates Hearing Threshold

If the test ear signal is crossing over and is heard in the non-test ear, thresholds are likely artificially low: You aren't yet measuring the test ear's threshold. With plateau masking, you will put in noise into the non-test ear, initially at a low intensity level – a level just 10 dB above the non-test ear threshold. If there was cross hearing, this noise level should elevate your measured threshold, but it may not be enough to eliminate all cross hearing. Figure 5-1 begins to illustrate.

Chapter 5. Air-Conduction Plateau Masking

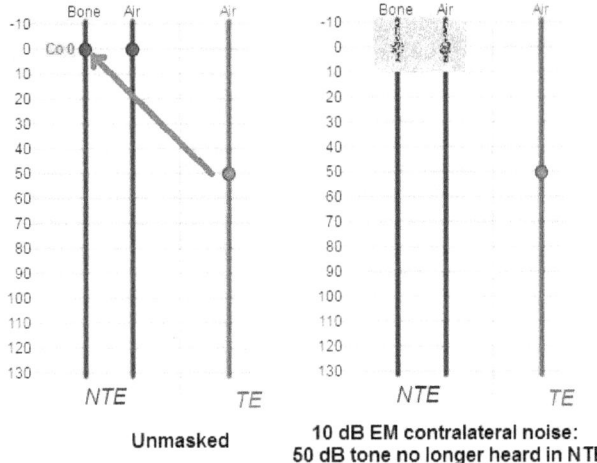

Figure 5-1. A person with unilateral hearing loss, who has 50 dB interaural attenuation (IA), is tested. The unmasked test ear threshold is 50 dB HL, the crossover (Co) is 0 dB HL, which is heard in the non-test ear by bone-conduction. On the right side of the figure, 10 dB EM of masking noise is put into the non-test ear. This masks the crossover. The patient would no longer hear the 50 dB HL tone presented to the test ear.

Example of the Plateau Approach to Masking

Let's examine the case where the true test ear threshold is 70 dB HL in a patient with unilateral sensorineural hearing loss. (In this first case, we will not show any central masking effect.) As was illustrated in Figure 5-1, without masking, the patient who has 50 dB interaural attenuation (IA) will detect the crossed-over tone when it is 50 dB HL: The 50 dB HL tone lost 50 dB as it crossed to the non-test ear cochlea. Because 0 dB HL is the bone-conduction threshold of the non-test ear, the crossed-over tone was heard. That crossover could be masked with as little as 0 dB EM, but in the first step of plateau masking, you start with the masking noise at 10 dB above the air-conduction threshold. As shown in 5-1, that prevents cross hearing of the 50 dB HL tone. But, with only 10 dB of noise in the non-test ear, we will not yet be able to accurately measure the threshold. When the signal level is raised to 65 dB HL, the crossover is 15 dB HL. That would be audible in the presence of 10 dB EM – the signal would "pop out" over the noise and be heard (Figure 5-2).

Chapter 5. Air-Conduction Plateau Masking

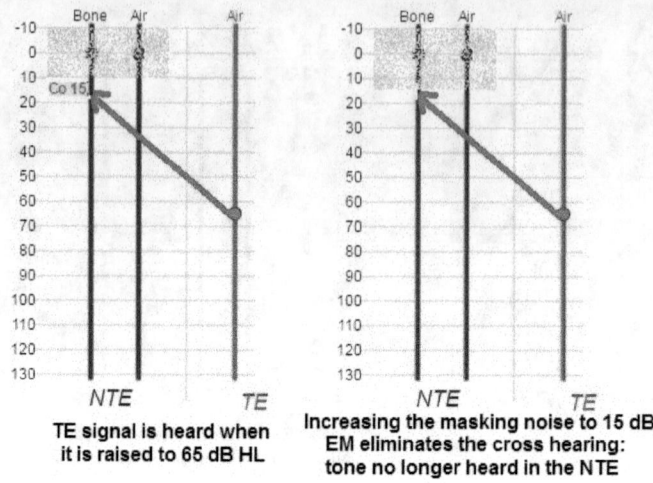

Figure 5-2. With 10 dB EM in the non-test ear, the measured threshold is 65 dB HL. This crossover will not be audible when the masking noise is raised to 15 dB HL.

If the noise is raised further, to 15 dB EM, the 65 dB HL test ear signal crossover will not be audible, and since that is below the test ear threshold, it is not heard in the non-test ear either. When the test ear signal is 70 dB HL it is heard in the test ear (because in our example, that was the test ear threshold). But note the 70 dB HL test ear signal is also crossing over and can heard in the non-test ear. Increasing the masking noise intensity another 5 dB will prevent the cross hearing, but the tone will remain audible in the test ear (Figure 5-3).

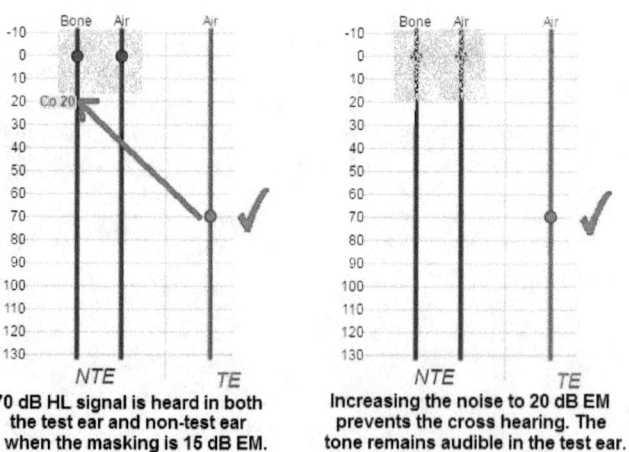

Figure 5-3. With 15 dB EM in the non-test ear, the crossed-over signal is heard. Increasing the masking noise to 20 dB EM eliminates the cross hearing. The patient is now hearing the signal only in the test ear and the threshold is accurately measured.

Chapter 5. Air-Conduction Plateau Masking

At this point, the noise can be increased again another 5 dB (or more, e.g. to 80 dB EM) and the same result will occur. The patient will hear the signal in the test ear and respond. The crossover is masked, so the NTE will not be stimulated. (Figure 5-4)

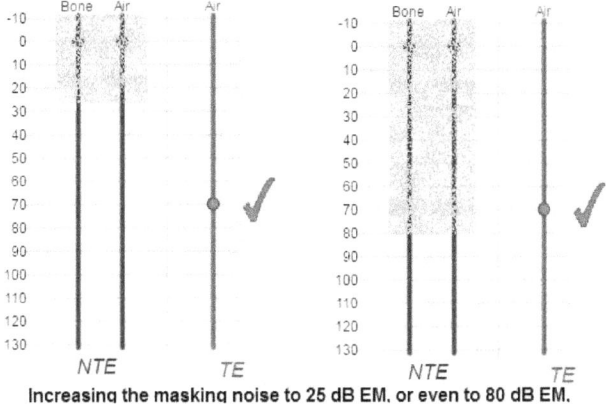

Increasing the masking noise to 25 dB EM, or even to 80 dB EM. does not alter the threshold since the crossover is already masked, and the test ear is responding to the signal.

Figure 5-4. Once the masking noise is adequate, increasing the noise levels modestly (e.g. to 25 dB EM, or even to 80 dB EM) has no further effect. The test ear threshold is the same. The masking noise is more than enough to prevent the crossover from being heard.

Overmasking Elevates Hearing Thresholds Artificially: Crossback Occurs

The masking noise cannot be increased indefinitely, however. When the noise in the non-test ear is sufficiently intense, the noise will cause a vibration of the skull, and that noise will **"cross back (CB)"** to the test ear, and prevent hearing of the test tone. This is called **over masking (OM)**. In Figure 5-5, 120 dB EM in the left ear loses 50 dB due to interaural attenuation. It is creating a right ear bone-conducted cross-back signal of 70 dB HL. The masking noise having crossed back will prevent hearing of the 70 dB HL threshold-level signal, and the test ear threshold increases. Each 5 dB increase in masking noise will increase the test ear measured threshold by 5 dB.

Chapter 5. Air-Conduction Plateau Masking

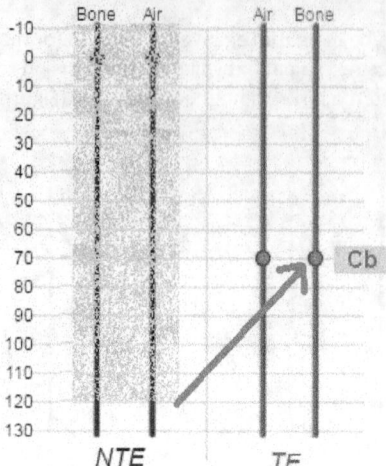

If 120 dB EM is put into the non-test ear, the crossback would be 70 dB EM, which is enough to prevent hearing the 70 dB HL threshold-level test ear signal. Overmasking is occurring, elevating the test ear threshold.

Figure 5-5. Overmasking occurs when the non-test ear noise level is intense enough to cross back (Cb) to the test ear and mask the test ear tone. The interaural attenuation value is the same as for crossover, in this example it is 50 dB. The crossback of the noise to the test ear elevates the measured threshold.

The Plateau in the Plateau Masking

If you plot the test ear threshold as a function of the contralateral noise level (as in Figure 5-6), you observe a period where each 5 dB increase in noise level causes a corresponding increase in threshold. This is the "undermasking" portion of the plateau masking procedure. As you increase the noise levels further you hopefully find the "plateau": a period during which increasing the masking noise level has no effect on threshold. The plateau ends when overmasking begins. You may not always see the undermasking "side" of the plateau function. In some cases, your initial masking level is enough to "put you on the plateau".

Chapter 5. Air-Conduction Plateau Masking

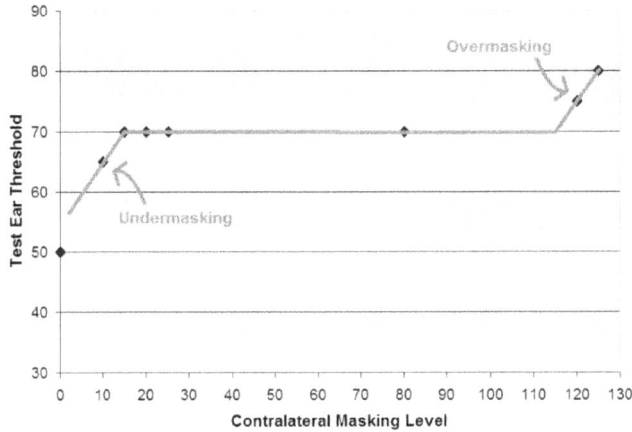

Figure 5-6. A diagram of the masking plateau showing the increase in threshold when the masking noise level is not sufficient, the plateau portion where increase in masking noise does not change threshold, and the overmasking portion, where each 5 dB increase in masking level causes a 5 dB increase in threshold. The plateau width in this illustration is from 15 to 115 dB EM – a 100 dB wide plateau.

Steps in the Plateau Masking Approach to Air-Conduction Masking

1. <u>Recognize the need for masking.</u> This implies that the non-test ear (better ear) has been tested first and the test ear's (poorer ear's) unmasked threshold has been obtained.

2. <u>Set the initial masking level at 10 dB above the non-test ear threshold. Re-obtain threshold.</u> In many cases, the threshold will shift due to either the initial threshold having been due to the signal crossing to the non-test ear, or if it was the test ear responding, the central masking effect may cause a slight elevation in threshold.

3. <u>Increase the masking in 5 dB steps, obtaining threshold each time.</u> Since increasing the masking noise will not improve the hearing threshold, you do not need to decrease the test signal intensity below the threshold obtained previously. If the tone is reliably heard at the previous threshold level, that is sufficient. (You don't need to use the full Hughson-Westlake technique.)

> Example: The right ear air-conduction threshold is 5 dB HL. The left ear unmasked air-conduction threshold is 70 dB HL. Masking is needed. The initial masking level is 15 dB EM. The threshold (measured in the left ear) is now 75 dB HL. The next step is to increase the masking 5 dB, to 20 dB EM. Rather than decreasing the stimulus level, determine if 75 is still heard. If it is, then the masking is increased another 5 dB, and threshold is again checked; but, if the 75 dB stimulus was not heard, then threshold would be re-established.

Chapter 5. Air-Conduction Plateau Masking

> 4▫ <u>Continue increasing the masking in 5 dB steps until three consecutive increases in the masking level occur with no change in hearing threshold.</u> As you are increasing the noise level, you might want to make a mental count "that was up once, that was up twice, that was the third time: done."

Examples of Plateau Masking for Air-Conduction

Example A: Non-test ear threshold = 5 dB HL

Masking level (dB EM) to NTE	TE Threshold (dB HL)
None	75
15	75
20	75 "up once" (first time increasing noise does not change threshold)
25	75 "up twice"
30	75 "up third time – done"

Example B: Non-test ear threshold = 20 dB HL

Masking level (dB EM) to NTE	TE Threshold (dB HL)
None	70
30	80
35	85
40	90
45	95
50	95 "up once"
55	95 "up twice"
60	95 "up third time – done"

A special circumstance occurs when the patient has no measurable hearing in the test ear. You don't need to continue to increase the masking noise intensity once you have reached the audiometer's maximum output level, and the patient no longer responds. Let's use the example of a patient with 80 dB interaural attenuation and a 10 dB threshold in the non-test ear. Masking would start with 20 dB EM in the nontest ear.

Chapter 5. Air-Conduction Plateau Masking

Example C: Non-test ear threshold = 10 dB HL

Masking level (dB EM) to NTE	TE Threshold (dB HL)
None	90
20	105
Note: the 10 dB SL of masking raised the threshold 15 dB. Why? There was a 5 dB central masking effect plus 10 dB elevation of threshold due to the masking noise.	
25	110
30	115
35	120
40	No Response

There is no need to increase the masking noise further – if there is no response with 40 dB EM contralaterally, then there will be no response with even more contralateral masking noise. (However, present the tone twice to ensure that it was truly not heard.) Mark the threshold with the "masked/no response" symbol. Testing at that frequency is done.

Note that clinically there is no need to determine the end of the plateau – you do not have to find the point where overmasking occurs. However, as we will discuss next, sometimes you will have a narrow plateau and sometimes you will find the point where overmasking begins.

Effect of Test Ear Conductive Loss: Narrowed Plateau Width (Overmasking Occurs at a Lower Level)

When there is conductive loss in the test ear, by definition bone-conduction is normal. This next section describes why this narrows the masking plateau; how the end of the plateau comes at a lower intensity level than if the loss is sensorineural.

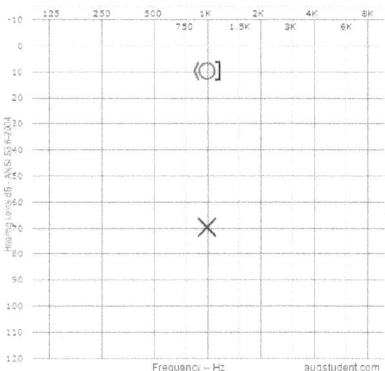

Figure 5-7. Typically, the bone-conduction threshold would not be known at this point in testing. You may be able to make the assumption that the loss is conductive based on the patient's history/symptoms, and if you have found abnormal immittance test results. In this case (Example D), masking is needed when testing air-conduction in the left ear. The initial masking level would be 20 dB EM, put into the right ear.

Chapter 5. Air-Conduction Plateau Masking

As shown in Figure 5-7, the left ear air-conduction threshold needs to be masked. This patient's right ear bone-conduction threshold is 10 dB, so this patient has an interaural attenuation of 60 dB. In this case, the true masked air-conduction threshold will be 75 dB HL. Let's next examine what would happen as we increase the masking noise levels.

Example D: Non-test ear threshold = 10 dB HL

Masking level (dB EM) to NTE	TE Threshold (dB HL)
None	70
20	75
25	75
30	75
35	75

At this point, we have increased the masking noise three times, and clinically, we would stop, marking the 75 dB HL masked threshold. How high could we go with the masking noise before we would overmask? To 70 dB EM. Recall that this patient has a 60 dB interaural attenuation value. Once the noise to the right ear reaches 70 dB EM, the cross back after the 60 dB IA will be 10 dB EM at the left ear cochlea. As shown in Figure 5-7, 10 dB HL is the test ear (left ear) bone-conduction threshold. The 10 dB EM crossback will prevent hearing of the 75 dB HL left ear air-conducted sound. Remember that this loss is conductive. The left ear air-conduction signal is 75 dB HL, the conductive loss attenuates the sound by 65 dB HL so that it is 10 dB HL at the test ear cochlea. The overmasking occurs at the level of the cochlea.

The plateau width is narrowed from what was shown in Figure 5-6, the case of unilateral sensorineural loss. In that example: the plateau started at 15 dB EM and ended at 115 dB EM – a 100 dB plateau width. In example D above, the plateau began at 20 dB EM and ends at 70 dB EM – there is a 50 dB plateau width. The end of the plateau is at a reduced intensity because of the normal bone-conduction threshold of the test ear; overmasking will occur at a lower intensity level than if the test ear has cochlear loss.

Effect of Non-Test Ear Conductive Loss: Reduced Plateau Width Due to Plateau Beginning with a Higher Intensity Masking Noise

Now, let's examine the complication of having conductive loss in the non-test ear (Figure 5-8). Let's again assume that the masked air-conduction threshold will be 75 dB HL, but this time, the loss is sensorineural in the left ear. The interaural attenuation is 60 dB in this example. Note that the non-test ear (right ear) has conductive loss with a 40 dB air-bone gap, and 50 dB air-conduction threshold. Again, the rule for starting the masking process is to use a level 10 dB above the non-test ear air-conduction threshold, so the starting masking level will be 60 dB EM in the right ear.

Chapter 5. Air-Conduction Plateau Masking

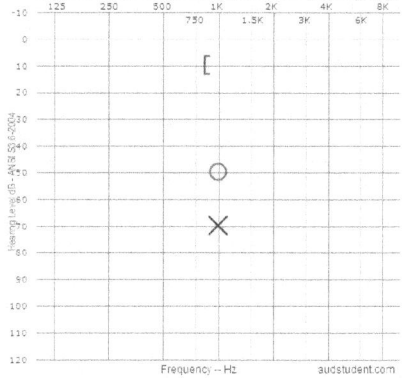

Figure 5-8. In this example, we examine the case of a patient who has right ear conductive loss and left ear sensorineural loss, with an eventual 75 dB HL air-conduction threshold.

The masking approach would be as follows.

Example E: Non-test ear threshold = 50 dB HL

Masking level (dB EM) to NTE	TE Threshold (dB HL)
None	70
60	75
65	75
70	75
80	75

This is our clinical "end point" – we would mark the threshold. Note that the patient had an unmasked left threshold of 70 dB HL and a right ear bone-conduction threshold of 10 dB HL, so the interaural attenuation is 60 dB HL. Since the test ear bone-conduction threshold in this example is 75 dB HL, the plateau would end at 135 dB HL (60+75). The plateau extended from 60 dB EM to 135 dB EM – a 75 dB plateau width.

Examine Figures 5-9 and 5-10. Note that in both the case of the test ear conductive loss (5-9) and non-test ear conductive loss (5-10), the plateau width is narrower than what was seen in Figure 5-6 where the test ear had sensorineural loss and the non-test ear had normal hearing. In that case, the plateau width was 100 dB HL. Figure 5-11 shows the three cases superimposed.

Chapter 5. Air-Conduction Plateau Masking

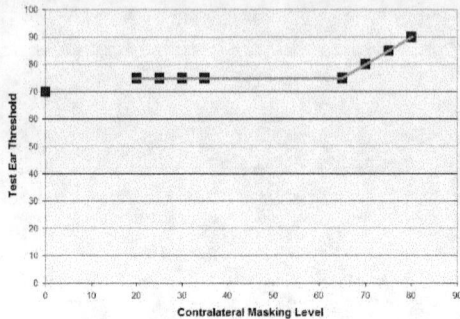

Figure 5-9. Masking plateau illustration in the case of test ear conductive loss. The end of the plateau is at a lower intensity. The plateau extends from 20 to 65 dB EM: The test ear conductive loss reduces the plateau width to 45 dB.

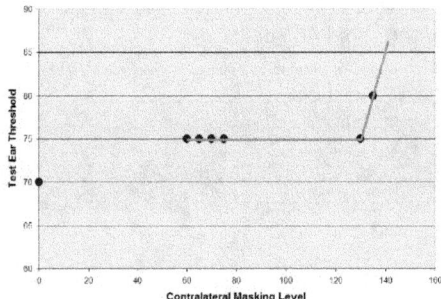

Figure 5-10. Masking plateau illustration in the case of non-test ear conductive loss. The start of the plateau is at a higher intensity. The plateau extends from 60 to 135 dB EM: The non-test ear conductive loss reduces the plateau width to 75 dB.

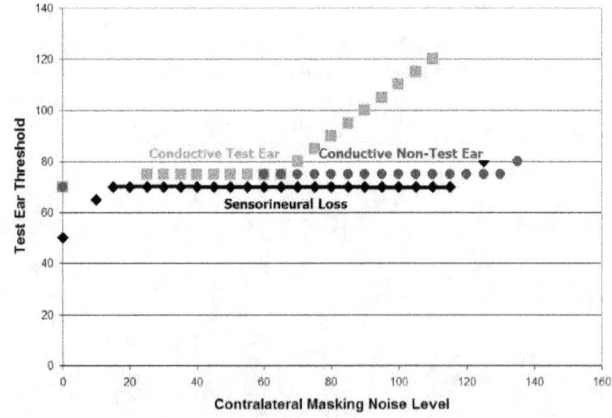

Figure 5-11. The three plateau charts superimposed. The point is that conductive loss, either in the test ear or non-test ear, will reduce the plateau width.

Chapter 5. Air-Conduction Plateau Masking

Effect of Bilateral Conductive Loss: Further Reduction in the Plateau Width

If the patient has conductive loss in each ear, the plateau width will be reduced "at both ends." The non-test ear conductive loss raises the intensity needed to "get onto" the plateau and the test ear conductive loss (normal bone-conduction hearing) means that the end of the plateau will be at a lowered level.

The example is shown in Figure 5-12.

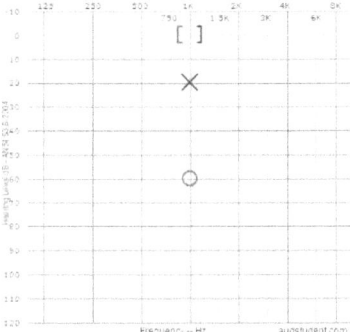

Figure 5-12. A case of asymmetrical conductive loss. The right ear air-conduction threshold requires masking. The true threshold for the right ear is 60 dB HL; however, the presence of contralateral masking evokes the central masking effect (listening with noise in the opposite ear is a more difficult task) and the right ear will have a masked air-conduction threshold of 65 dB HL.

Let's assume once again that this patient has a 70 dB air-conduction interaural attenuation value. The signal is not crossing over at an audible level; however, you don't know this, so you plateau mask. Masking would begin at 30 dB EM (10 dB above the left ear's air-conduction threshold.)

Example F: Non-test ear threshold = 20 dB HL

Masking level (dB EM) to NTE	TE Threshold (dB HL)
None	60
30	65 (due to the central masking effect)
35	65
40	65
45	65

Here's where we would conclude our testing. But let's continue to raise the masking noise level to see the overmasking portion.

50	65
55	65
60	65
65	65

Chapter 5. Air-Conduction Plateau Masking

This hypothetical patient had a test ear bone-conduction threshold of 0 dB HL and 70 dB interaural attenuation for air-conduction, so once the masking is 70 dB EM, you will begin to overmask. To continue . . .

70	70
75	75
80	80

As illustrated in Figure 5-13, the plateau width (from 30 to 65 dB EM -- 35 dB) is narrow.

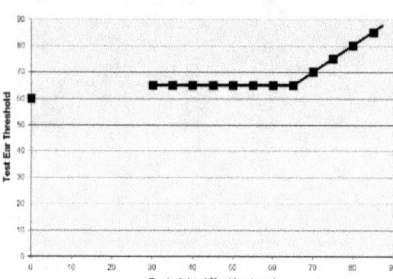

Figure 5-13. Effect of minor non-test ear conductive loss and concomitant test-ear conductive loss on the masking plateau. This patient has 70 dB interaural attenuation. The plateau portion is narrowed but present.

Masking Dilemmas: Plateau Cannot Be Found

There are times when a masking plateau cannot be found. Masking is needed, but as soon as masking is used, overmasking occurs.

Let's increase the non-test ear conductive loss size in the next example of a patient who has 60 dB of air-conduction interaural attenuation.

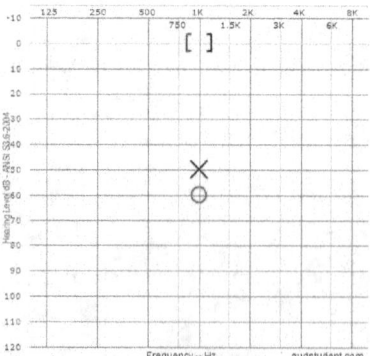

Figure 5-14. A masking dilemma example. The right ear air-conduction threshold requires masking. (Yes, so does the left ear.) The true threshold for the right ear is 60 dB HL; however, the presence of contralateral masking evokes the central masking effect

Chapter 5. Air-Conduction Plateau Masking

(listening with noise in the opposite ear is a more difficult task) and the patient will have a masked threshold of 65 dB HL. The case uses an interaural attenuation value of 60 dB.

In this case, the true threshold remains 60 dB HL, although it would be measured as 65 dB HL due to the central masking effect.

The masking approach would be as follows.

Example G: Non-test ear threshold = 50 dB HL

Masking level (dB EM) to NTE	TE Threshold (dB HL)
None	60

As masking is not yet used, the tone is heard in the test ear, but it is also crossing over because the interaural attenuation is 60 dB: The tone is heard bilaterally.

60	65

At this point, masking has eliminated the cross-hearing of the 60 dB HL tone, and the test ear's threshold is raised 5 dB due to central masking. Although the 65 dB HL tone is crossing over to the non-test ear, it is only at 5 dB HL and the masking is 10 dB above the non-test ear threshold, so the crossover is not audible. The 60 dB of contralateral masking noise would cross back at 0 dB HL, but the test ear tone is audible because it was increased 5 dB above the unmasked level due to the effect of central masking. Continuing with the plateau approach procedures, the masking noise is increased 5 dB, to 65 dB EM.

65	70

The 65 dB EM in the non-test ear is now interfering with hearing the tone in the test ear; the crossback level to the test ear cochlea is 5 dB HL. The test ear tone needs to be 10 dB above threshold, 70 dB HL, so that when it loses 60 dB due to the right ear air-bone gap, it is audible above the 5 dB EM crossback noise. As per the procedures for plateau masking, the noise is increased again.

70	75

Each increase in the masking noise level requires the test ear tone to increase by 5 dB in order to be audible above the crossback noise level, which increased 5 dB. The process continues. (Also see Figure 5-15.)

75	80
80	85
85	90
90	95
95	100
100	105
105	110
110	115

Chapter 5. Air-Conduction Plateau Masking

115	120
120	No response at audiometer output limit of 120

Failure to find a masking plateau leaves one uncertain. Is this indication of bilateral conductive loss and a patient who is untestable due to the masking dilemma, or does the patient have a unilateral profound hearing loss?

Note if Figure 5-14 that the left ear threshold is 50 dB HL, and that means that the left ear air-conduction threshold also needs to be masked: there is potential for crossover to the right cochlea. When plateau masking is attempted for the left ear, again there will be a masking dilemma. Since you can't have one or both ears with moderate/moderately severe conductive loss without masking and then have accurate results that show that both ears have profound loss with masking, you will be alerted to the presence of the masking dilemma.

That point merits repeating. If you start out with an audiogram that shows one or both ears has hearing, and with masking now find two "dead ears," that's an indication that you have come across a masking dilemma. Further, the cross-test principle will assist you. Immittance test results will be abnormal with bilateral conductive loss. Masking dilemmas occur with bilateral conductive loss.

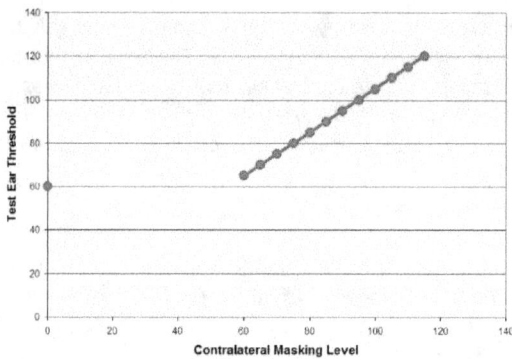

Figure 5-15. When a masking dilemma is present, there is no masking plateau.

Clinical Tips and Hints

Reduced Plateau Widths

If the plateau is narrowed, but has not entirely disappeared, you have a "narrowed plateau width." For example, if you turn the masking noise up twice (or even once) and threshold remains stable, but then threshold increases with each subsequent increase in the masking noise, you have a narrowed plateau width. I would recommend retesting to ensure that it is truly a narrow plateau and not a false positive response. If you are confident that you have a narrow plateau, then mark the results accordingly. If you are manually recording the audiogram, the standard notation is an asterisk by the threshold, and corresponding footnote of "reduced plateau width." With a computerized audiometer, you would need to write a comment listing those ear/frequency/transducer combinations with reduced width plateaus.

Chapter 5. Air-Conduction Plateau Masking

Use Deeply Inserted Earphones Bilaterally

When TDH headphone use was standard, masking dilemmas were more common. Air-conduction interaural attenuation values are lower with TDH supra-aural headphones. Insert earphones provide greater interaural attenuation, especially in the low frequencies where the conductive loss is usually worst. If you ensure that the inserts are deeply seated – that the foam is level with the entrance of the meatus or in even more deeply and not definitely visibly protruding – you will cause the interaural attenuation to be even higher and reduce the likelihood of having a masking dilemma.

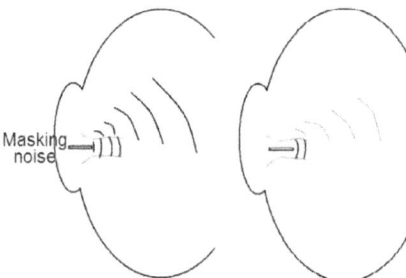

Figure 5-16. Inserting the insert earphone more deeply reduces the area of the external auditory meatus that is vibrating, which reduces the interaural attenuation. Deep insertion reduces crossover and crossback, which reduces the likelihood of experiencing a masking dilemma.

Avoid Presenting the Test Tone Immediately After Increasing the Noise Level

Plateau masking can be tedious: increase the noise, present the tone, increase the noise, present the tone . . . If your timing between increasing the noise and presenting the tone is predictable, you greatly increase the risk that the patient will give false positive responses. It is also possible that the patient (e.g. a young child) will become confused and begin to think that the desired response is to signal you when the noise increases. Even if the patient is not confused, anticipation of the tone coming right after the noise increase promotes false positive responses. Vary your timing: occasionally use a mere second between noise increase and tone presentation, other times wait several seconds. This way you can be alerted to the false positive response (when the patient responds before you present the tone.)

Using mQuest

mCalc is not for use in determining the initial masking level. It helps you determine the formula masking level – the one level to use to mask the crossover (the topic of this e-book, chapters 7-10.) mQuest levels 6 and 7 test your skills at setting the initial masking levels.

Chapter 5. Air-Conduction Plateau Masking

Using AudSim Flex© to Practice Plateau Masking

The AudSim Flex© software program includes example masking patients. This is a separate program from mCalc and mQuest. It is available for purchase at the bargain price of $19.99 at audstudent.com. There are tutorials on this website about how to install and use the software.

Although the software has a "Threshold Assistant" mode for unmasked testing, we have not yet implemented "Masking Assistant". This feature is planned for an upcoming version, but it has been planned for a long time now. I may have to retire before I have a chance to do that.

Key Concepts

Steps in the plateau procedure for air-conduction testing

- Recognize the need for masking.

- Set the initial masking level at 10 dB above the non-test ear threshold. Re-obtain threshold.
- Increase the masking in 5 dB steps, obtaining threshold each time.
- Continue increasing the masking in 5 dB steps until three consecutive increases in the masking level occurs with no change in hearing threshold.

Conductive loss in either the test ear or in the non-test ear narrows the masking plateau width. Bilateral conductive loss narrows the plateau further, and in some cases there is no plateau. If you cannot find a plateau for a patient with bilateral conductive hearing loss, you have what is termed a "masking dilemma" — masking is needed, but the use of masking causes overmasking.

Chapter 6

Plateau Masking for Bone-Conduction Testing

Quick Reference – BC Plateau Masking Steps

- Masking is needed if there is a 15 dB or greater difference between the test ear air-conduction threshold and either the unmasked NTE or TE bone-conduction threshold.
- The initial masking level = NTE threshold + 10 dB pad + OE. Where recommended occlusion effect text values for insert earphones are.

> 250 Hz - 20 dB
> 500 Hz - 10 dB
> 1k Hz - 5 dB

It is acceptable to omit the OE values when the non-test ear has an existing conductive loss equal to or greater than the OE size.

- Increase the NTE noise until three consecutive 5 dB increases do not increase the TE threshold.
- If unmasked testing shows bilateral conductive loss, and masked testing shows both ears are "dead", then it is a masking dilemma.

Overview

The process of plateau masking for bone-conduction testing is similar to what is done with air-conduction plateau masking. The only difference is that the occlusion effect needs to be considered.

The Occlusion Effect

The occlusion effect is an increase in the amount of bone-conduction sound entering the cochlea when that ear is covered (occluded). This occurs when you are masking because we must cover the non-test ear in order to deliver the air-conduction masking noise. The masking noise level needs to be increased in order to compensate for this normal, additional increase of the bone-conducted sound into the non-test ear cochlea. The exception to the rule that you need to account for the occlusion effect when testing bone conduction is if the non-test ear has significant conductive hearing loss. If the conductive loss is larger than or equal to the size of the occlusion effect, the occlusion effect can be omitted. (Technically, you can reduce the occlusion effect amount by the size of the NTE air-bone gap, but let's not "go there" right now. It will be a topic for formula masking,Chapter 9.)

How the Occlusion Effect Occurs: Enhancement of the Bone-Conduction by Air-Conduction Route of Bone-Conduction Hearing

There are three ways in which vibration of the skull during bone-conduction testing creates movement of cochlear fluids: the distortion of the cochlea shell, the inertial lag of the stapes footplate in the oval window, and the bone-conduction by air-conduction mechanism. Only the latter is relevant to the discussion of the occlusion effect. If you would like a review of the other mechanisms, let me shamelessly plug my textbook,The Hearing Sciences (2nd edition, authored by Hamill & Price, available from Plural Publishing).

When the bone oscillator, placed on the mastoid, creates sound, it vibrates the skull, including the portions of the temporal bones that the external auditory canals run through. This creates a vibration of the walls of the ear canals, which creates an air-conducted signal. When the ear is not occluded, the pressure wave mostly exits the ear canal; though some energy goes inward, vibrating the tympanic membrane. As shown in Figure 6-1, when the ear is covered (e.g. by the insert earphone in the right ear) the sound is channeled into the middle ear (being unable to escape the outer ear.)

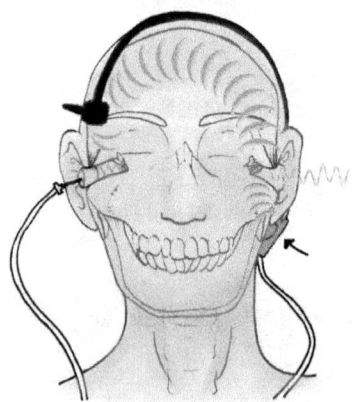

Figure 6-1. The bone-conducted sound vibrates the head, including the ear canals, which creates an air-conducted sound. When the ear is not occluded (left ear, with the bone oscillator), this air-conducted sound will escape. However, the non-test ear is occluded with an insert earphone. The bone-conducted sound that has become an air-conducted signal is funneled into the middle ear. Because the right ear in this illustration is occluded, the sound has greater intensity at the right ear cochlea (which receives the combination of the bone-conduction crossed over signal and the "bone-conduction by air-conduction" part). Artwork by Heather Marinello.

Chapter 6. Bone-Conduction Plateau Masking

The Size of the Occlusion Effect Depends on the Transducer Used

Why the Occlusion Effect is Larger with Supra-Aural Headphones

If a supra-aural headphone is used, e.g. a TDH series 39, 49, or 50 headphone in MX-41/AR rubber cushions, the vibration of the bony and cartilaginous areas of the external meatus, the vibration of the cartilage of the pinna, and even some vibrations of the side of the head are channeled inward towards the tympanic membrane and the occlusion effect is large. If you use an insert earphone, only the medial portion of the ear canal vibrations create sound, which is then funneled into the middle ear. Therefore, insert earphones create a lowered occlusion effect size. (Refer back to Figure 2-1 for an illustration.)

<u>Demonstration of the Occlusion Effect and How It Changes With Type of Earphone/Headphone Used</u>

Next time you are in the clinic/lab, send a low-frequency sound to the bone oscillator (e.g. 500 Hz at 40 dB HL). Put the bone oscillator on your forehead (slip the metal band around the back of your head). Put an insert earphone in one ear and note the increase in the sound level. Now put the TDH headphone over the other ear, and you will notice how much louder the sound is in that ear.

But, you probably aren't in the lab as you read this, so here's another way to demonstrate and help you remember the concept that the occlusion effect is greater with supra-aural headphones, or any whole-ear occlusion. Hum a low-pitch note. Yes, this creates an air-conducted sound, but it also vibrates your nasopharyngeal area (back of your throat and nose), which creates a bone-conducted sound: You've set your entire skull into vibration since all the bones of the head are fused. (You may even feel some of that vibration in your chest.) Keep humming at a steady volume and push your tragus in to occlude the one ear. You should hear your voice more loudly in that ear now. Now create a cup shape with your other hand – make sure it's pretty air tight – and place that over your entire pinna (other side of the head) while still occluding the other ear with tragal compression. This should give you even greater bone-conduction by air-conduction enhancement – it sounds louder in the cupped ear.

A trait common to professors is the desire for complete scientific disclosure, though sometimes that lessens a good example. Note that I had you occlude your tragus first, and then cup your other ear. This gives you a bilateral occlusion effect, which is greater than a monaural one. You can alternate between occluding a single ear with tragal occlusion and your cupped hand; that will still demonstrate the concept, it's just not as dramatic. Or, with the ears both occluded, one with each method, concentrate – where do you hear the hum as louder? It should be the cupped-occluded ear (if you have a nice tight cup over the ear). But I digress.

<u>A Digression on Forehead Bone Oscillator Placement</u>

As long as I'm digressing -- a note on forehead bone-conductor placements. While mastoid bone oscillator placement is common, some clinics use a forehead placement. Although the bones of the adult head are fused, and one usually concludes there is no interaural attenuation, you will obtain different (worse, higher dB level) thresholds with a forehead placement if your audiometer is calibrated for mastoid placement. The advantage is that you can leave the oscillator in place; it does not need to be repositioned as you switch between masking the right and left ears. The symbol used (^) denotes "best bone-conduction threshold" to the audiogram reader, eliminating an ambiguity for those who

Chapter 6. Bone-Conduction Plateau Masking

are testing bone conduction only once on a patient with symmetrical sensorineural loss. (You don't have to choose either record the unmasked right or left ear symbol.)

I have seen use of a shortcut, particularly in those who use the forehead vibrator placement. The audiologist places the insert earphones in each ear and leaves them there as the audiologist switches between left and right bone-conduction threshold testing. This means that the test ear is occluded, and will have thresholds enhanced by the occlusion effect size. So, it's worthwhile to think about the occlusion effect: What is its average size, what's the minimum and maximum you would expect to see? What is the effect of using this shortcut? You'll see in just a little bit that it varies considerably from person to person.

The Presence of the Occlusion Effect Means that the Initial Masking Level Must be Increased

When you cover the non-test ear with an earphone or headphone, that causes an occlusion effect: the bone-conducted sound that has crossed over to the non-test ear has increased in intensity at the non-test ear cochlea. This means that when we start plateau masking, the initial masking level needs to be raised to compensate for the increased bone-conducted sound in the non-test ear. The question is "How much more air-conducted masking noise is needed in the non-test ear?" Obviously, that depends on the transducer used to deliver the masking noise.

The Size of the Occlusion Effect for TDH Headphones

In the early days of audiology, testing was conducted with TDH-style headphones. Early research fully explored the size of the occlusion effect. Common recommended values if using **TDH headphones** were:

250 Hz -- 30 dB
500 Hz – 20 dB
1000 Hz – 10 dB

These values represent the AVERAGE occlusion effect values. That's interesting, given how cautious audiologists have been traditionally. Those who have a greater than average occlusion effect will have a louder sound at the non-test ear, and require a greater masking noise level. This is unlikely to be a concern if you are plateau masking where you will add in the average occlusion effect size and add an additional 10 dB that I'll call the "safety pad" to your initial masking level. Unless the occlusion effect size were 25 dB more than expected (the 15 dB plateau width plus the 10 dB "safety pad"), one would still observe a shift in the masked threshold as the noise level increases, if the occlusion-effect-enhanced tone were crossing over. The size of the occlusion effect is more of a concern when testing using a formula approach, where one level is assumed to be enough to mask the occlusion-effect-enhanced crossover. (Formula masking is the topic of the remaining chapters.)

Chapter 6. Bone-Conduction Plateau Masking

The Size of the Occlusion Effect for Insert Earphones

Other Texts Recommend an Average Insert Earphone Occlusion Value – Not a Conservative Value

Texts recommendation insert earphone occlusion effect values that are based on average values. The common recommendations are:

> 250 Hz – 10 dB
> 500 Hz – 0 to 10 dB
> 1000 Hz and above – 0 dB

These values are acceptable when plateau masking, but *I cannot recommend them if formula masking.* Since the hope is that you will eventually use formula masking, the sections below review why these values are not "safe enough" for formula masking, and the argument will be made for use of these values:

> 250 Hz – 20 dB
> 500 Hz – 10 dB
> 1000 Hz – 5 dB
> 2000 Hz and above – 0 dB

Research Studies on the Size of the Occlusion Effect for Insert Earphones: No Consensus and High + 2 Standard Deviation Values

Let's examine available data on the average and largest expected occlusion effect values seen clinically. There has been surprisingly little research related to insert earphones.

Table 6-1. Dean and Martin (2000) reported these occlusion effect values, obtained using 20 young normal-hearing females (mastoid bone oscillator placement). The mean, and the values 1 and 2 standard deviations (SDs) above the mean are shown. Recall that ~84% of patients will have occlusion effect values at or below the +1 SD level, and virtually all will have levels at or below the +2 SD values. The -2 SD range shows the minimum expected. Values are rounded.

	250 Hz Shallowly inserted earphone	250 Hz Deeply inserted earphone	500 Hz Shallowly inserted earphone	500 Hz Deeply inserted earphone	1000 Hz Shallowly inserted earphone	1000 Hz Deeply inserted earphone
Mean	16	9	10	6	6	1
+1 SD	23	15	15	12	12	4
+2 SD	29	21	19	17	18	8
(SD)	7	6	5	6	6	4
-2 SD	+3	-3	1	-5	-6	-6

Chapter 6. Bone-Conduction Plateau Masking

In the past I had students do a class assignment in which they measure the occlusion effect of their lab partner: Measure the bone-conduction thresholds first without occlusion and then again with occlusion of the non-test ear. Obviously, this was not testing conducted with the same level of experimental control as seen for Dean and Martin.

Table 6-2. Results of NSU class assignment to measure the occlusion effect. n=68.

	250 Hz	500 Hz	1000 Hz	2000 Hz	4000 Hz
Mean	10	6	6	1	2
+1 SD	19	13	13	6	7
+2 SD	28	20	20	11	12
SD	9	7	7	5	5
-2 SD	-8	-8	-8	-9	-8

The average values are similar to what Dean and Martin reported for deeply inserted earphones, except that 1000 Hz shows a greater occlusion effect value.

One additional study merits review. Stenfelt and Reinfeld (2007) measured the increase in ear canal sound pressure levels from shallow occlusion (inserting 7 mm (about 0.3 inches) into the meatus, and of deep (22 mm, about 0.9 inches) insertion. Their "shallow" seems shallower than typical, and their deep insertion is deeper than what one would use clinically. An interesting variation in their methods was that they measured the sound level increase in the ear canal, as well as testing audiometrically. Their values are for occlusion of the ipsilateral ear (oscillator on same side as the ear being occluded, while the contralateral ear was masked with a well-vented insert earphone.)

Chapter 6. Bone-Conduction Plateau Masking

Table 6-3. Stenfelt and Reinfeld (2007) recorded the increase in sound pressure levels in the ear canal (measured) and those obtained using threshold testing evaluations with insert earphones (threshold). Data interpolated from figures. N=20.

	250 Hz Shallowly inserted earphone	250 Hz Deeply inserted earphone	500 Hz Shallowly inserted earphone	500 Hz Deeply inserted earphone	1000 Hz Shallowly inserted earphone	1000 Hz Deeply inserted earphone
Measured						
Median	28	12	12	-4	8	-5
Maximum	45	30	22	9	12	5
Threshold						
Median	22	10	13	0	10	-2
Maximum	35	25	30	15	22	12

Figure 6-2 gives a graphic illustration of these data. As we compare across the three sets of studies, we see that the mean or median value for deeply inserted earphones support the conventional text book recommended occlusion effect values of

> 250 Hz – 10 dB
> 500 Hz – 0 to 10 dB
> 1000 Hz and above – 0 dB.

But – the question remains. Should we use the average occlusion effect size, or the worst-case scenario values – the largest occlusion effect you are likely to encounter?

Chapter 6. Bone-Conduction Plateau Masking

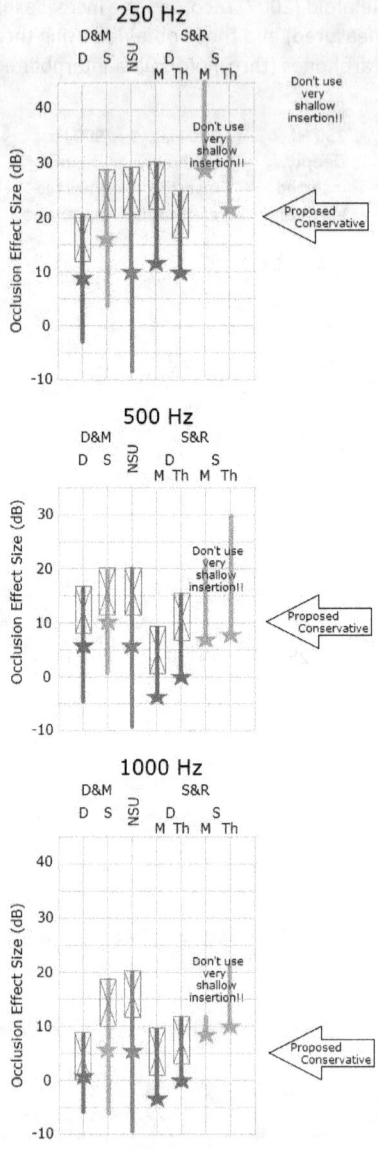

Figure 6-2. Data from Dean and Martin (2000) (D&M), from the NSU student assignment, and from Stenfelt and Reinfeld (2007) (S&R). D indicates deep insert earphone insertion and S denotes data when the inserts had a shallow insertion depth. Stars show the mean, and the vertical bars show the range of data. As will be discussed below, the very highest of the range need not be used. The arrow to the side of the figure shows the value recommended. Note that the mean data are in agreement with other text's recommended occlusion effect values.

Chapter 6. Bone-Conduction Plateau Masking

The Occlusion Effect Values You Choose Depend on How Conservative You Want to Be

If we use the median/mean values, we need to understand that half of our patients will have a greater occlusion effect. If we use values based on deep insertion of the insert earphone and position the insert earphone shallowly in the patient's ear, we will further under-estimate the occlusion effect.

With plateau and formula masking, some cautiousness is already in effect – we typically use 10 dB more masking than what we calculate as a minimum amount desired (the 10 dB pad). This helps to compensate for minor masking calibration errors, a shallow insert earphone insertion, or a larger than average occlusion effect size. But, the argument can be made that it is possible to have both a masking calibration error and a large OE value, in which case using the average occlusion effect value and the 10 dB safety "pad" is not sufficiently cautious.

<u>Test-Retest Variability Inflates the Maximum Occlusion Effect Size</u>

Should we always use the maximum possible interaural attenuation value, just as we use the minimum interaural attenuation value in deciding when to mask? Probably not, and here's why. The maximum values probably are inflated by some measurement error. There is general agreement that there is NOT an occlusion effect for the high frequencies (although Stenfelt and Reinfeld (2007) occasionally measured one – but, in situ SPL level measurements are not necessarily immune to error, so it's hard to say what that means). Notice from Table 6-2 (data from my students' labs) that occlusion effects as high as 12 dB can be found in the high frequencies. It's likely that's not really an occlusion effect, but instead it is the result of test/retest variability. If, by chance, the measured unoccluded bone-conduction threshold was 5 dB lower than the true value, and the occluded bone conduction threshold were 5 dB higher than the patient's real threshold, that would give an artificial 10 dB occlusion effect. I expect that test/retest variability is affecting the low-frequency +2 standard deviation range as well: The upper range of occlusion effect values comes partially from test/retest measurement error.

Next, examine the "negative two standard deviation" value. There should be no negative value of an occlusion effect, yet we see about 8 dB can happen because of this test/retest variability (Tables 6-1 and 6-2). Thus, my recommendation. Ignore the "top 8" dB of the two standard deviation range - - assume that comes from test/retest variability. This lowers the recommended occlusion from the rather high levels one would have to use if the maximum values were applied.

<u>Using Too High an Occlusion Effect Value Creates More Overmasking Risk</u>

There is a danger in assuming that the occlusion effect is higher than it truly is – presenting more masking noise will create more problems with overmasking, so using the most conservative positive value may not be a good idea. How cautious should one be then?

A Somewhat Data-Based Recommendation on Conservative Occlusion Effect Values

Figure 6-3 and Table 6-4 show the occlusion effect values that the text will suggest, which are based upon the suggestion of using 8 dB less than the maximum or +2 SD value from the studies.

Chapter 6. Bone-Conduction Plateau Masking

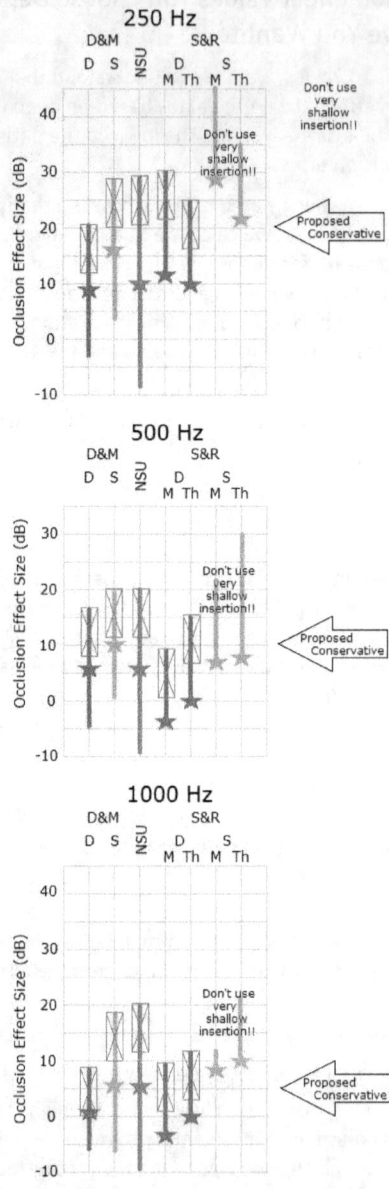

Figure 6-3. *(deja vu)* The "proposed conservative" values come from an average across studies of the occlusion effect value that is about 8 dB below the maximum or + 2 SD values. The data from shallow insertion data from Stenfelt and Reinfeld are omitted, as those insertions were extremely shallow. Abbreviations: D&M = Dean and Martin (2000) (D&M), NSU = NSU student assignment, S&R = Stenfelt and Reinfeld (2007). D indicates deep insert earphone insertion and S denotes data when the inserts had a shallow insertion depth.

Table 6-4. A fairly cautious range of occlusion effect values (in dB), based on the discussion above (that assumes a deeply inserted insert earphone). The four values in the top row come from Tables 6-1, 6-2 +2 SD values, and each of the maximum deep insertion SPL and threshold measurements from Table 6-3 – with 8 dB then subtracted from these values. The 8 dB correction downward is an attempt to reduce influences of test/retest measurement error on the maximum values observed across the studies.

	250 Hz	500 Hz	1000 Hz
+2SD or maximum values minus 8 dB	12,20,22,17	9,12,1,7	0,12,-3,4
Average of the four values	18 dB	7 dB	4 dB
Rounded Up	20 dB	10 dB	5 dB

Summary of Occlusion Effect Values One Could Use

Table 6-5. Various potentially supportable occlusion effect values are shown in this table. As illustrated, the other text recommendations and the mean occlusion effect values are substantially lower than what some patients may experience, even with deeply inserted earphones, which is why you may want to use a higher occlusion effect value.

	250 Hz	500 Hz	1000 Hz
Other texts recommend	10	0-10	0
Average of the four values	10	5	0
+1 SD approximate values	15-20	10-15	10
"Fairly cautious" (aka "proposed conservative") recommended values	20 dB	10 dB	5 dB

As shown in the table above, the mean occlusion effect values are a bit lower than what I recommend, particularly for formula masking where you have to anticipate the amount of sound at the non-test ear with fairly good accuracy.

The mCalc software and mQuest game that accompanies this book default to the "fairly cautious" recommended values, but allows you to put in other values if you prefer. (The audiometer simulator – AudSim – has the patient's occlusion effect values in the patient profiles; you cannot alter them.)

The Occlusion Effect Can Be Omitted If There is Significant Conductive Loss

In order for the occlusion effect's bone-conduction by air-conduction enhancement to occur, the additional energy needs to pass through the tympanic membrane and middle ear. If there is significant conductive loss, then the occlusion effect is lessened or eliminated. Therefore, if testing a patient with conductive loss in the non-test ear, if that conductive loss is equal to or larger in magnitude than the occlusion effect size, you can omit the step of adding in the occlusion effect. Chapter 9 covers this concept in greater detail.

Steps in the Plateau Masking Approach to Bone-Conduction Masking

1. Recognize the need for masking. To review from chapter 3, masking is needed if there is an air-bone gap, or the concern that there could be an air-bone gap (the unmasked bone-conduction threshold is 15 dB or more better than the test ear air-conduction threshold).

2. Set the initial masking level at the non-test ear air-conduction threshold, plus 10 dB, plus the occlusion effect size. This book will use 20 dB at 250 Hz, 10 dB at 500 Hz, and 5 dB at 1000 Hz.

3. Increase the masking in 5 dB steps, obtaining threshold each time if threshold increases.

4. Continue increasing the masking in 5 dB steps until three consecutive increases in the masking level occur with no change in hearing threshold.

Example of Bone-Conduction Plateau Masking

Let's examine masking in a case of unilateral sensorineural hearing loss. Examine Figures 6-4 and 6-5

Chapter 6. Bone-Conduction Plateau Masking

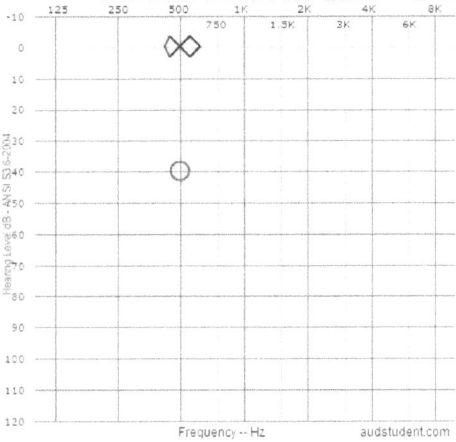

Figure 6-4. Bone-conduction masking example of testing the right ear at 500 Hz. The patient's occlusion effect value is 10 dB. The right ear loss is sensorineural.

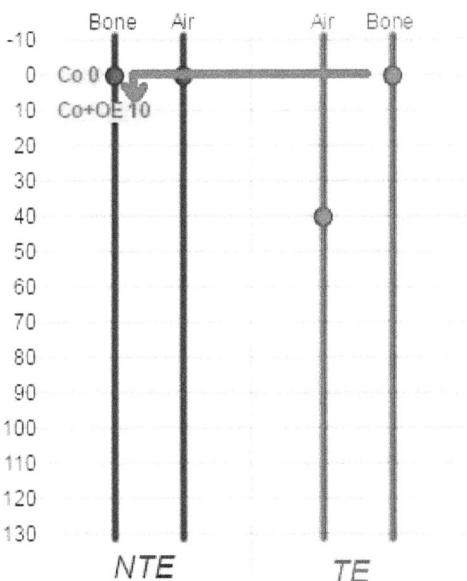

Figure 6-5. Bone-conduction interaural attenuation is 0 dB so the entire right ear bone-conducted signal crosses to the non-test (left) ear. When the non-test ear is occluded, the crossed over bone-conducted sound (Co) is increased to 10 dB HL (Co+OE).

To mask the right ear 500 Hz threshold in Figure 6-4 and 6-5, we would begin with the masking noise at 20 dB EM (0 dB left ear threshold + 10 dB safety pad + 10 dB occlusion effect).

Chapter 6. Bone-Conduction Plateau Masking

Example:
Masking level dB EM	Threshold dB HL
None	0
20	15

Note that although the test ear tone is 15 dB HL, which crosses to the non-test ear at 15 dB HL, the occlusion effect enhances the tone by 10 dB, making it 25 dB HL at the non-test ear cochlea and therefore audible above the 20 dB EM. (Figure 6-6).

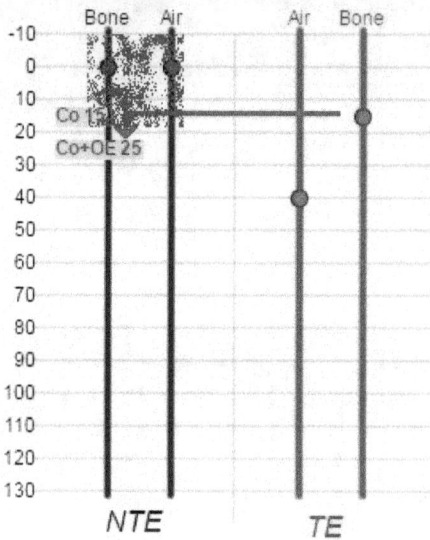

Figure 6-6. The 20 dB EM raised the test ear bone-conduction threshold to 15 dB HL.

In our example, the test ear true threshold is 40 dB HL, so the 15 dB HL bone-conduction signal is not yet heard in the test ear. As the masking noise is increased, threshold will increase proportionally.

Masking level dB EM	Threshold dB HL
25	20
30	25
35	30
40	35
45	40

The tone is now heard in the test ear, so the threshold will no longer increase with increases in contralateral masking noise levels.

50	40 "up once"
55	40 "up twice"
60	40 "up a third time- done"

Chapter 6. Bone-Conduction Plateau Masking

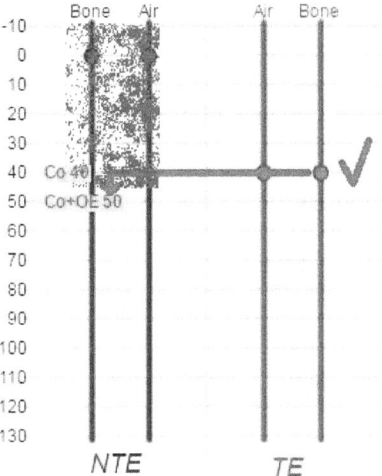

Figure 6-7. The 40 dB HL bone-conducted signal to the right ear was stimulating both by the right and left ears when the masking level was 45 dB HL.

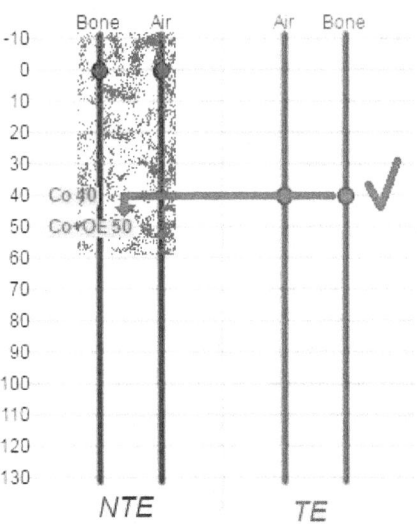

Figure 6-8. Increasing the noise to 60 dB HL prevents the cross-hearing. The threshold remains 40 dB HL because it is being heard in the test ear.

Figures 6-7 and 6-8 show that we are "on the plateau" as the noise increases from 45 to 60 dB EM. In this case of unilateral sensorineural hearing loss, the masking noise can be increased to a very high level before overmasking would occur. If the patient has an 80 dB interaural attenuation value (an average value for 500 Hz), then overmasking would occur when the noise was at 120 dB EM (80 dB above the 40 dB HL test ear threshold). See Figure 6-9.

Chapter 6. Bone-Conduction Plateau Masking

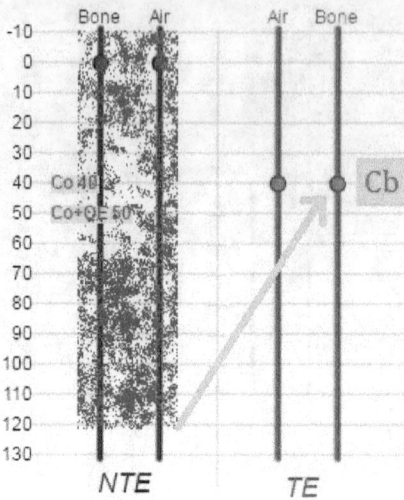

Figure 6-9. The 120 dB EM air-conducted masking to the left ear loses 80 dB as it crosses back (Cb) to the test ear (this patient has 80 dB air-conduction interaural attenuation). The 120 dB EM would prevent audibility of the test ear tone – overmasking would occur.

Effect of Test Ear Conductive Loss: Overmasking Occurs at a Lower Level

Just as is true with air-conduction masking, having conductive loss in the test ear narrows the plateau width. By definition, bone-conduction thresholds are normal if the test ear has conductive loss. The patient with an 80 dB air-conduction interaural attenuation value will experience over masking once the non-test ear masking noise is 80 dB above the test-ear bone conduction threshold. (If the test ear bone conduction threshold is 5 dB HL, 85 dB EM will cause overmasking.) However, since the test ear bone-conduction thresholds are normal, you will find that you "step onto" the plateau at a low intensity level.

Effect of Non-Test Ear Conductive Loss: Reduced Plateau Width Due to Plateau Beginning with a Higher Intensity Masking Noise

When the non-test ear has conductive loss, the initial masking level must be higher to overcome the loss. Since plateau masking starts at 10 dB above the non-test ear threshold, the start of the bone-conduction masking plateau will be raised, which narrows the plateau.

Effect of Bilateral Conductive Loss: Further Reduction in the Plateau Width

Just as was true for air-conduction masking, bilateral conductive loss further reduces the plateau width when testing bone-conduction. You have both the narrowing of the plateau width that is caused by starting at a higher masking level intensity due to the non-test ear conductive loss and you have the threat of overmasking when the sound crosses back to the normal test cochlea.

Chapter 6. Bone-Conduction Plateau Masking

If you add in the occlusion effect (recall, it is not needed with significant conductive loss in the non-test ear), then you would start with higher masking levels, causing even further narrowing the plateau since it means starting masking at a higher intensity level.

Masking Dilemmas: Plateau Cannot Be Found

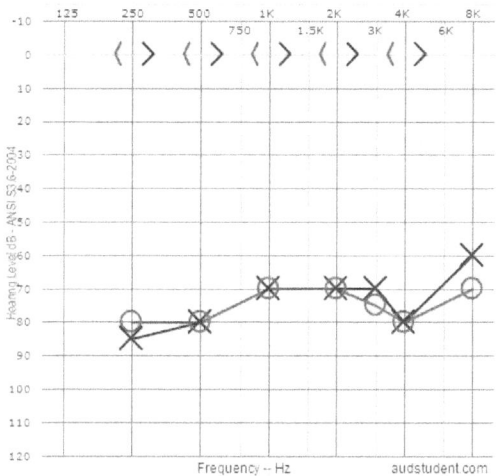

Figure 6-10. An audiogram that illustrates a typical bilateral "maximum conductive loss" when testing with insert earphones.

While historically the maximum conductive loss was said to be "50-60 dB," this was what was found when testing with supra-aural headphones. If testing with insert earphones, more loss may occur. A case where no sound is sent through the middle ear, a true maximum conductive loss, is shown in Figure 6-10, which reflects fairly average interaural attenuation values for insert earphones. (Remember that the AC signal, once it is loud enough to create skull vibration, stimulates both the test ear and non-test ear cochleas. This creates the "maximum" conductive loss.) If masking is attempted, as soon as the contralateral noise is loud enough to be audible and begins to mask the cross-over, the masking noise will cross back. Each 5 dB increase in the masking noise causes a 5 dB threshold elevation. Eventually, the results of bone-conduction testing will be no response at the output limits of the audiometer, as shown in Figure 6-11. If you initially have a loss in one or both ears that is moderately severe or worse, and then after masking have "two dead ears," then you have experienced a classic masking dilemma. The reason the test results show no hearing when masking is that overmasking raised the thresholds.

Chapter 6. Bone-Conduction Plateau Masking

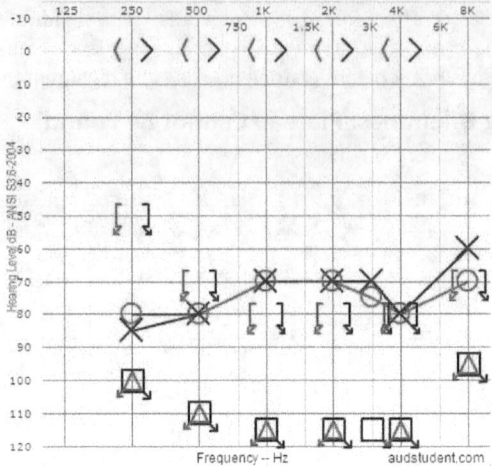

Figure 6-11. Illustration of the results of attempting masking when there is a masking dilemma. Test results show two ears with profound sensorineural hearing loss, a result that does not make sense given that unmasked testing indicated hearing in one or both ears.

Clinical Tips and Hints

The Maximum Conductive Loss Typically Seen is Not a True Maximum Conductive Loss

What would have to happen to have sound by-pass the middle ear entirely? A middle ear with a congenital abnormality such as being filled with bone – that would do it!

Let's review the concept of impedance mismatch for sound transmission to the middle ear. If there were no middle ear, if the oval window functioned as the tympanic membrane, then sound would lose about 30 dB of energy because of the impedance difference of the cochlear fluid versus air. (Remember that the function of the middle ear is to increase the sound pressure through the mechanical advantage primarily coming from the collection of sound at the relatively large tympanic membrane, and the funneling of that sound into the small area of the stapes footplate.)

Sometimes conductive loss creates a situation that is worse than just the loss of the normal impedance matching transformer. Consider a break in the ossicular chain at the incudo-stapedial joint. In order to vibrate the cochlear fluids, sound has to be loud enough to vibrate the tympanic membrane which has the additional mass of the malleus and incus resting on it. The sound billowing into the middle ear is not directed just to the stapes. The sound has to be intense enough to move the stapes-laden oval window.

But even in the case of a break in the ossicular chain, the conductive loss will still allow some sound transmission inward through the middle ear. The vibrating air inside the middle ear would have to move the stapes. That's hard to do, but it is doable.

It is typical for conductive losses not to be much worse than 50-60 dB HL, which corresponds to the old TDH earphone "maximum conductive loss." But that's not to say it's a true "maximum" conductive loss.

Chapter 6. Bone-Conduction Plateau Masking

Why this lengthy discussion? As a reminder that many times you can mask a moderate bilateral conductive loss successfully – if the loss is not truly maximum, if the air-conducted sound is not by-passing the middle ear – then you may be able to successfully plateau mask.

Omit the Occlusion Effect with Significant Conductive Loss

As mentioned previously, when bilateral conductive loss is suspected (i.e. air-conduction hearing loss bilaterally and abnormal immittance), if you are not able to plateau mask with inclusion of the occlusion effect values, try omitting them. They are not needed if the conductive loss size is equal to or greater than the occlusion effect size. This lowers the needed masking noise level, and if the loss is not quite "maximum conductive" you may be able to establish masked thresholds. The plateau width may be reduced to 10 dB, but if that plateau is repeatable, it is acceptable.

Test High-Frequency Bone Conduction First If You Expect a Masking Dilemma

You may want to start bone-conduction testing at 4000 Hz when faced with a challenging bilateral conductive loss. Conductive losses are typically of smallest magnitude in the high frequencies, and at 4000 Hz the minimum interaural attenuation for air-conduction testing (which determines when crossback will occur) is 60 dB HL; the average is 80 dB HL, and it is possible to have a value as high as 100 dB at this frequency. Even a narrow plateau at some frequencies will help ascertain if cochlear sensitivity is asymmetrical.

Document "Reduced Plateau Width" Appropriately

Remember to document situations where your plateau width was less than 15 dB but repeatable and reliable as "reduced plateau width" test results. A reliable (repeatable) 10 dB plateau would be enough to know that you are measuring the test ear hearing; however, the additional documentation helps those reviewing the testing or trying to replicate your results.

mQuest Game Practice and AudSim

mQuest Levels 8 and 9 provide practice at determining the initial masking level to use. If there is significant conductive loss in the non-test ear, the game requires you to remember to omit use of the occlusion effect. Immittance test results are given to help you make the decision. For those who have not yet studied immittance, abnormal results are consistent with conductive pathology. The test ear immittance results are also shown, but that is irrelevant to your decision making.

The audiometer simulator (AudSimFlex) allows you to practice plateau masking for bone-conduction testing.

Chapter 6. Bone-Conduction Plateau Masking

Key Concepts

The steps in the bone-conduction plateau masking approach are as follows:

- Recognize the need for masking.

- Set the initial masking level at the non-test ear air-conduction threshold, plus 10 dB, plus the occlusion effect size. This book recommends using 20 dB at 250, 10 dB at 500 Hz, and 5 dB at 1000 Hz.
- Increase the masking in 5 dB steps, re-obtaining threshold if threshold shifts.
- Continue increasing the masking in 5 dB steps until three consecutive increases in the masking level occur with no change in hearing threshold.

Conductive loss in either the test or non-test ear has the effect of narrowing the plateau width, and with bilateral conductive loss, you may face a masking dilemma: Masking is needed due to air-bone gaps bilaterally, but when masking is applied, it causes overmasking.

The occlusion effect will not occur when there is significant conductive loss in the non-test ear, so when facing a potential masking dilemma due to bilateral conductive loss, omit the occlusion effect values when attempting to plateau.

Chapter 7

What is Formula Masking and Why Use It?

Formula Masking

Formula masking predicts what the masked threshold will be, determines how much masking is needed, and uses this one level of masking noise. When plateau masking, the noise increases in 5 dB steps. In contrast, in formula masking the goal is for one calculated level to be used, without adjustment. However, if your estimate of threshold is not correct, you will have to adjust the masking intensity. Formula masking is more time efficient.

Plateau Masking is "The Standard," But It Can Be Time Consuming

Plateau masking is the "gold standard" of masking. If you found the unmasked threshold, used the appropriate initial masking level, increased the masking level 15 dB, and the threshold has not changed with those three 5-dB increases, you are assured that you have masked correctly.

However, in cases of unilateral severe / profound hearing loss, plateau masking takes a long time. Consider the case of bone-conduction testing of a unilateral "dead" ear when the better ear has a 0 dB threshold. The unmasked 2k Hz threshold is likely 0 dB HL. Assume that the NTE air-conduction threshold is normal. You would start with 10 dB of masking, which probably elevates the bone-conduction threshold to 20 dB HL (10 due to peripheral masking and 5 dB increase from central masking, and the signal needs to be 5 dB above the noise to be heard). Each time you increase the non-test ear noise in 5 dB steps, the threshold increases in 5 dB steps.

This process is repeated until the bone-conduction signal level is at the audiometer maximum, i.e. 75 dB HL. Most likely, the contralateral noise is 75 dB HL at the time you obtain the no-response. Masking levels used were 10, 15, 20, 25, 30, 35, 40, 45, 50, 55, 60, 65, 70, 75.

To ensure that the patient didn't anticipate the tone and respond just due to the increase in the masking noise level, the audiologist also had to test at a slow rate, pausing after turning up the noise by a variable amount of time to ward off false-positive responses. And heaven forbid that the patient is one prone to false-positive responses! Finding one threshold can take several minutes. There is a faster way!

Formula Masking Defined

When conducting formula masking, the audiologist puts a calculated amount of noise into the non-test ear to prevent cross hearing.

There is more than one way to formula mask. The audiologist may formula masked based on the initial unmasked threshold, but to be time efficient, the audiologist considers that the threshold will likely shift once masking is used and base the calculations on that expected threshold. There are other variations to the formula masking approach. The audiologist can determine the highest level of masking noise that can be used, and/or the minimum level that is needed, use either of those levels, or put in a level somewhere between that minimum and the maximum level.

The audiologist may need to make an adjustment to the noise level – e.g. if it was predicted that the loss was moderate and threshold testing is showing greater hearing loss, the masking noise may need to be increased; or vise-versa, if the assumption was that the loss was profound, and thresholds are coming in better than expected, the audiologist may need to decrease the noise level – if the high noise level could have overmasked. But relatively few masking level intensity adjustments (if any) are made when using a formula masking approach. This offers a time savings.

Formula masking requires some thinking, but it becomes easier and easier with practice. The audiologist will always be thinking about what signal levels could be crossing to the non-test ear, and what masking noise level is needed to mask the crossover. An additional consideration is needed – whether using a loud noise in the non-test ear could be uncomfortably loud.

Another concern is that if the masking noise is intense enough, it too can vibrate the skull and create cross-hearing. In the case of **overmasking**, the crossed-back-to-the-test ear sound interferes with hearing the test ear signal.

Formula masking means thinking about how much crossed over, and then finding a masking noise level that is enough to mask the cross over, but not so loud that it is uncomfortable or could overmask. With that one level of noise in the non-test ear, threshold is found. If threshold was what you expected – what you based your calculations on – you are done! No up 5, up 5 . . .

Once the basics of hearing testing are mastered, it is enjoyable to have the mental challenge of figuring out how much masking is needed, and fun to see introductory-level audiology students' looks of amazement when the audiologist seemingly uses intuition in nearly automatically setting the masking level to "the" level needed. But reaching that zenith takes a bit of time and effort. Why put forth the effort? Keep reading.

Time is Money, Fast is Good

Increasing your test efficiency means seeing more patients, but it also maximizes your diagnostic results. Whether testing children or adults with limited mental capabilities, cooperation with testing occurs only for a limited amount of time. Being efficient can mean the difference between complete and incomplete test results.

Patients appreciate short test times. While taking a hearing test is not difficult, it does require attention. It's a rare patient who would want to have a larger number of test tones to detect. Formula masking saves both you and the patient time.

Sometimes You Cannot Plateau; You Must Formula Mask

When conducting word recognition testing, you cannot plateau mask. Increasing the masking noise and determining if the word recognition score stayed the same or improved or worsened wouldn't work – word recognition scores vary from list to list even at the same intensity. It's not feasible to determine if the scores are changing meaningfully as the contralateral noise level is adjusted. Also, it would be time consuming and tedious.

When estimating hearing thresholds using auditory brainstem response (ABR) testing, one has to be as efficient as humanly possible in order to obtain the needed thresholds. Repeating testing with varying levels of contralateral noise is out of the question. The audiologist has to know how much noise to use to mask any possible crossover of the test signal to the non-test ear. Routine use of a formula masking approach during pure-tone testing is the best way to ensure that you are able to mask during ABR testing, which is a situation that involves concentration on many things in addition to masking.

There is No Single Way to Formula Mask, But All Approaches are Based on the Same Constructs

The profession of audiology has not adopted one single formula for air-conduction masking testing, nor one for bone-conduction masking. As a result, each professor/clinical preceptor may want their students to use a slightly different approach. That's the bad news. The good news is that all the approaches are based on the same underlying ideas.

- How intense was the crossed over signal?
- Is that crossed-over signal audible in the non-test ear?
- How intense does the masking noise need to be in order to mask the crossover?
- What level of noise would be the most I can use before the noise will cross-back and be heard in the test ear?

It sounds harder than it really is. We will take it a step at a time, and in the next chapter, we begin with air-conduction formula masking. You have already worked on the first steps if you have completed the mQuest learning game, levels 1 through 9, the plateau masking games

An Audiologist Has to Know His/Her Test Technique's Limitations!

There are occasions where the audiologist wants to mask using a formula, but in making the mental calculations, determines that the minimum level is either at or close to the maximum that can be safely used without cross-back interfering with the test ear hearing the signal, or sometimes those calculations tell you the impossible: The minimum to use is already above the maximum to use without concern or reservation. In those cases, the audiologist reverts to plateau masking if that is an option. (So, please don't replace your understanding of how to plateau with how to formula mask – you need to know both!)

Chapter 7 – Why Formula Mask?

Key Concepts

- Formula masking uses a single masking level, although the masking noise level may be adjusted a few times if the test ear threshold is not what was expected.

- It is more time efficient than plateau masking.

- However, there are times when formula masking creates too many uncertainties, and the audiologist reverts to plateau masking.

Chapter 8

Formula Masking for Pure-Tone Air-Conduction Testing

Quick Reference: The Formulae

These formulae are listed at the start of the chapter to make the book a better reference. Skip to the next section if you are a first-time reader.

Minimum Masking Level

Minimum Masking Level (MMin) =
TE signal level – IA + significant NTE ABG + 10 dB
(or if you prefer)
For insert earphones :
  TE signal level – 40 dB + NTE ABG
For supra-aural phones :
  TE signal level – 30 dB + NTE ABG

"Signal Level" is your estimate of the eventual, masked threshold, not the un-masked threshold.

Maximum Masking Level

Maximum Masking Level (MMax) =
BC threshold of the TE + IA – 5
(which is)
For insert earphones : BC TE + 45 dB
For supra-aural phones : BC TE + 35 dB

Term "Effective Masking" Level

Audiometers are calibrated so that the noise signals are in decibels of effective masking (dB EM), not dB HL. dB EM is defined as the intensity of a noise that masks the same dB HL level signal.

An example is worth more than the formal definition. When establishing the standards for dB EM, a two-channel audiometer was used. The noise and the pure tone were routed to the same earphone. The masking noise level in dB SPL was adjusted until it just masked the pure tone. For example, a 2000 Hz 40 dB HL tone was masked by 49 dB SPL of narrow-band noise (remember – routed to the same earphone). The audiometer is then calibrated so that 49 dB SPL narrow-band noise is produced when the audiologist presents 40 dB EM. (In contrast, the pure tone level of a 40 dB HL tone is 43 dB SPL for insert earphones.)

Chapter 8 – Formula Masking – Air-Conduction

X dB EM Masks a Crossed-Over Bone-Conduction Signal of X dB HL

Any time you produce x dB EM, it masks x dB of signal presented to the same ear (if your audiometer is calibrated correctly).

The dB EM calibration reference is convenient. It means that if an air-conducted signal crosses over to the non-test ear (NTE) cochlea at some level, for example, 25 dB HL, then if we can put 25 dB EM (or more masking) into the non-test ear cochlea, then we will have masked the crossover.

It's really as simple as that! To figure out the theoretical minimum level you will need to use, you would

> a) Determine how intense the crossover could be. Ex: test ear (TE) signal is 60 dB HL using insert earphones. The crossover will be 10 dB HL if the patient has that minimum interaural attenuation value of 50 dB.
>
> b) Input, at a minimum, enough masking noise so that it reaches the cochlea at 10 dB EM (higher is OK as long as overmasking does not occur). In practice, you would want a bit more (at least 10 dB more) in case there is a calibration error with your noise level.

Minimum Masking Concepts

Compensate for Non-Test Ear Conductive Loss

The presence of conductive loss in the non-test ear means that air-conducted masking is reduced in intensity as it travels through the outer and middle ear systems. To make sure that you have enough noise at the cochlea, you have to overcome any conductive component.

Estimate the Size of the Air-Bone Gap or Decide that a Non-Test Ear Air-Bone Gap is Unlikely

Conducting immittance testing before audiometry is a good way to determine if you may need to add an estimate of the size of the non-test ear conductive loss to your masking calculations. If the non-test ear had normal tympanograms, and even more importantly, present ipsilateral reflexes, then it's a safe bet that the ear has sensorineural loss. You don't need to add in an air-bone gap estimate in calculating the minimum masking level.

Patient symptoms, otoscopic evaluation, and audiogram shape also can lead one towards or away from suspicion of conductive loss. This first section will focus on the minimum level of masking that is needed; we will then think about the maximum level. If you are unsure of whether there may be conductive loss, you can opt to use a masking level that is closer to the maximum than it is to the minimum. If you use the "maximum approach" you don't have to have a perfect estimate of the conductive loss size.

The safest assumptions will be to consider the worst case scenario when there is evidence of conductive loss (e.g. abnormal tympanometry and absent reflexes): make the

Chapter 8 – Formula Masking – Air-Conduction

calculations as if the loss in the non-test ear IS conductive. If the calculations indicate that masking may cause overmasking, then don't formula mask: plateau mask.

After you obtain the entire audiogram, you will want to do one last review of your masking levels. If you had used a minimum masking approach, and if a conductive hearing loss component was present when you had not anticipated it, you'll need to test again with more masking noise. (But the total test time may still be less than if you had plateau masked.)

"Significant" Air-Bone Gap

Add in the air-bone gaps only if they are "real." Remember that there is a 5 dB test-retest variability to hearing threshold testing, so, once you are finished with all your testing, if you notice the occasional 5 or 10 dB air-bone gap, don't be concerned. You will be adding in a 10 dB safety pad – using 10 dB more masking than the absolute minimum, so this will help if there are small air-bone gaps. I would recommend adding in air-bone gaps of 15 or higher. It is safer to add in the air-bone gap than omit it, so if you are "auditing" your final test results before taking the patient out of the booth, if you have any question that there was insufficient masking, add in those air-bone gaps to your formula and re-test the air-conduction thresholds that are in question. Air-conduction testing uses a 50 dB IA value in the formulae, and most patients have a much greater IA, so for air-conduction testing, it's not so critical that you consider minor air-bone gaps. When we move to bone-conduction testing, then it is important. You don't have the overly-cautious interaural attenuation value to mitigate against the probability of undermasking.

Minimum Masking Air-Conduction Formula Process

To formula mask when testing via air-conduction, you ask:

<u>1) Could the AC signal cross over to the non-test ear?</u>

This thought generally doesn't even need to enter your mind until the air-conduction test signal level is 50 dB or higher. (More on that in the next section.) You next asked yourself:

<u>2) Could the crossed-over signal be heard by the non-test ear cochlea? How intense might that the crossed over signal be?</u>

This requires thinking about the bone-conduction threshold of the non-test ear, since crossover happens when the air-conducted sound vibrates the skull and creates bone-conducted sound.

Example: at 1000 Hz we have:
Left ear AC threshold = 70 dB HL
Right ear   = 10 dB HL
The 20 dB cross over (assuming use of insert earphones with a 50 dB interaural attenuation) could be heard.

<u>3) Add the estimated NTE air-bone gap to the crossover level.</u>

Is there conductive loss in the non-test ear (NTE)? If so, what is the largest size it could realistically be? Add the estimated NTE air-bone gap to the crossover level. The noise presented by air conduction will lose intensity (in the amount of the air-bone gap size) as it

Chapter 8 – Formula Masking – Air-Conduction

passes through the outer and middle ear. To ensure it is at the desired level when it reaches the cochlea, it has to be increased by the size of the NTE air-bone gap.

> **Example:** at 1000 Hz we have:
> Left ear AC threshold = 70 dB HL
> Right ear = 10 dB HL
> If immittance is normal, and there are no symptoms of conductive loss, then I would not add any estimated air-bone gap size to my formula.
>
> If instead this adult patient had abnormal immittance, I would consider that the bone-conduction threshold may be 0 dB.
> I will add 10 dB to my formula.

There is just one more step to finding the minimum masking level.

<u>4) Add 10 dB more for safety</u>

I call this a "pad" or "safety pad." If my estimate of the air-bone gap is slightly low, or if the masking noise is slightly off calibration, or if there was a small unrecognized non-test ear air-bone gap, this extra little bit of noise reduces the likelihood that I will undermask.

> **Example:** at 1000 Hz we have:
> Left ear AC threshold = 70
> Right ear AC threshold = 10 dB HL.
> Immittance is normal
> **The total formula: MMin = TE signal level – 40 + NTE ABG.**
> Above, the steps were to:
> take the signal level, subtract 50, then add 10 as a safety pad,
> Which simplifies to : signal level – 40.
>
> Formula = Signal level – 40 + NTE ABG.
>   = 70 – 40 = 30 dB EM
> If immittance had been abnormal, to mask the 70 dB signal I need:
>   (70 - 40 + 10) = 40 dB EM

> Min. Masking total formula for insert earphones:
> MMin = TE signal level – 40 + NTE ABG.

There's a Limit to Prudent Caution

When determining the need for masking and estimating the air-bone gap and setting the mimimum level, you may ask yourself whether it is appropriate to assume that bone conduction is better than 0 dB HL. For example, could a 45 dB HL pure tone cross over and be heard if the bone-conduction threshold is -5 dB? If the patient is a child, this may be appropriate. Or if estimating non-test ear air-bone gap size, should you consider that perhaps the bone-conduction score is really -5 or -10 dB HL? Again, you can if it is a child.

How cautious you want to be depends on you and your preceptor's general approach. You can be cautious from the start and make these super-conservative assumptions (particularly if it's a child). You could also "play the odds" – assume that the patient will be

Chapter 8 – Formula Masking – Air-Conduction

typical (bone-conduction threshold not better than 0 dB HL). After you have completed testing both ears, your last step should be to see if you failed to mask when masking was needed, or didn't sufficiently account for a small air-bone gap. If either is the case, you would just retest with sufficient masking.

However, remember that the assumption of a 50 dB interaural attenuation is already a very conservative assumption, (unrealistically so for low-frequency pure tones.) In reality, the minimum interaural attenuations are higher – refer back to Chapter 2, Figure 3. That means that the amount of masking you are using, which was based on the 50 dB IA number, is higher than you probably need. And if you find a low-frequency asymmetry of 50 dB between the test ear air-conduction threshold and the non-test ear bone-conduction threshold, in reality, it is not truly crossover. (In the 1000 to 3000 Hz range, the IA could be as low as 50 dB.)

Review of the Formula for Minimum Masking Level

Let's review the formula, using the abbreviations:

Mininum Masking Level (MMin) =
   TE AC signal level – IA + NTE ABG + 10 dB.

For insert earphones this is:
   TE AC signal level – 40 + NTE ABG

For TDH earphones this is:
   TE AC signal level – 30 + NTE ABG

Estimate Eventual Threshold – Use as "TE AC Signal Level" in the Min. Masking Formula

The test ear hearing threshold is likely to shift once masking is introduced, due to the initial results being due to cross-hearing, or due to the central masking effects. For this reason, using a minimum level of masking, based upon the unmasked threshold, isn't a good idea.

When threshold shifts (as it likely will, even if just 5 dB due to central masking), then you would have to re-calculate the minimum level and adjust the masking noise. That would be as inefficient as plateau masking. How would you estimate the eventual test ear threshold?

- If you believe that the test ear is "dead," you would base your minimum masking formula on the audiometer's maximum output level (e.g. 125 dB HL)
- If you are retesting a patient, estimate that the threshold is now 20 dB worse than the last time you tested (or more, if you have reason to suspect greater shift.)
- If you find an umasked threshold and expect thresholds to shift once masked, calculate the minimum masking level based on the assumption that the eventual, masked threshold will be 20 to 40 dB above the unmasked threshold level.

Maximum Masking Level Before Overmasking (MMax)
Overmasking: NTE AC Noise Crosses Back to TE via BC

Setting the minimum masking level ensures that you are not undermasking – that the non-test ear is prevented from hearing the crossed-over signal. It is equally important to make sure that the presence of masking noise in the non-test ear is not crossing back resulting in overmasking.

The interaural attenuation for masking noise is the same as it is for pure tones (i.e. a minimum of 50 dB for insert earphones). For example, a noise level that is 70 dB EM could cross back to the test ear cochlea at 20 dB EM. As with crossover, the crossed-back signal is sent via bone conduction. This means we need to compare the crossed-back noise level to the TEST ear BONE-conduction threshold.

Calculating Maximum Masking Level

To determine the maximum level of noise to safely put into the non-test ear without concern for overmasking, estimate the best (lowest dB number) TEST ear bone-conduction threshold that is reasonably expected, add the interaural attenuation, then subtract 5 dB. Why subtract 5 dB? If the dB EM at the cochlea is exactly equal to the pure tone level, you will have over masking. You need to reduce the masking level 5 dB to find the maximum level of noise that can be used without risk of overmasking.

Maximum Masking Level MMax = TE BC threshold + IA − 5 dB
For insert earphones, this simplifies to :
   TE BC threshold + 45 dB
And for supra-aural earphones:
   TE BC threshold + 35 dB

The maximum level is often very high. Let's examine the case of an 80 dB HL sensorineural loss. The maximum masking level that can be used before overmasking with insert earphones is 80 + 50 − 5: 125 dB EM.

Use the "Best Reasonable" BC Threshold when Calculating MMax

For air-conduction minimal masking levels, you are advised to estimate that the test ear air-conduction threshold will come in at least 20 dB higher than the unmasked threshold. Don't do that when thinking about the bone-conduction threshold. You need to consider the "worst case scenario" – that is, the best bone-conduction threshold you are likely to find. If immittance was normal and the patient symptoms are pointing away from any conductive involvement, then I would use the unmasked air-conduction threshold as my estimate of the bone-conduction threshold. (I may not get a full 2 out of 3 Hughson-Westlake threshold before masking, but I'll use that as the approximation of threshold.)

If you want to be particularly cautious, you can estimate that the bone-conduction threshold will be even lower (e.g. 10 dB lower).

Use the Cochlear Sensitivity if the BC Threshold will be "No Response" or Vibrotactile

To make it easier to read the formula, I am writing "BC threshold" in formulae, but really what I mean is cochlear sensitivity. For example, if the air-conduction threshold is 90 dB HL, and the audiometer bone-conduction output limit is 70 dB HL, use the 90 dB HL number in the formula.

If you predict that, when you are conducting bone-conduction testing, you may find vibrotactile thresholds, again, think about cochlear sensitivity when calculating MMax – not the "threshold that is probably feeling not hearing."

Estimating the Test Ear BC Threshold if Conductive / Mixed Loss is Suspected

If immittance test results are abnormal for the test ear, then the air-conduction threshold does not predict the bone-conduction threshold. The only thing you can safely do is assume the entire loss is conductive.

(Well, if you had a prior audiogram with masked bone-conduction results, that could be an exception to the rule that you have to consider that the entire loss could be conductive. Use the prior bone-conduction threshold in that case (it's unlikely that cochlear sensitivity has improved significantly since you last tested the patient.))

Formula masking is easiest and safest for sensorineural losses – if estimating the TE or NTE air-bone gap is too uncertain, and/or the air-bone gaps are large – then plateau masking is preferable. Formula masking still works when there are minimal air-bone gaps, even in each ear. Just remember the saying: "When in doubt, plateau it out."

Don't Create Loudness Discomfort!

Using the maximum level instead of the minimum masking level is efficient – it will eliminate having to turn up the masking noise if the hearing threshold is higher than what you used in your calculation of the minimum masking level. However, the maximum level may be very high, and you don't want to cause your patient discomfort. In the example of 80 dB unilateral sensorineural loss, MMax was 125 dB EM. Putting 125 dB of effective masking noise into the normal-hearing non-test ear would be painful.

Even with hearing loss in the non-test ear, the MMax level may cause loudness discomfort. If the patient has asymmetrical hearing loss, with profound cochlear loss in the test ear (e.g. poorer ear sensorineural loss of 110 dB HL and better ear threshold 50 dB HL), while you could use effective masking levels that are as high as the audiometer output limits without fear of overmasking, loudness grows quickly in ears with sensorineural loss. A UCL of 100-110 dB HL would be expected for the non-test ear with 50 dB of cochlear loss. Don't use levels near MMax if it would be uncomfortable (unless you are required to do so to reach MMin.)

If you don't have experience in estimating UCLs, there's an app for that too, and that app is currently free (PC or Mac OSX platforms). It's called Andros and found on at www.audstudent.com/andros. You can estimate MCL (most comfortable loudness level) and UCL (uncomfortable loudness level) for various hearing losses, sensorineural and those with conductive components.

Chapter 8 – Formula Masking – Air-Conduction

Formula Masking Ideally Uses ONE Level of Noise!

To be most efficient, you would like to input a noise level to the non-test ear that doesn't require adjustment as you establish the test ear threshold. Using the maximum masking noise level, based on the best-possible test ear bone-conduction threshold you expect, would do that; however, as discussed above, it may recommend very high noise levels, and using those levels would not make you popular with your patients.

This is where different audiologists / preceptors take different approaches. Some will advocate something near the maximum level, moderated as needed to avoid loudness discomfort. (But, as we will soon discuss, if you use MMax, you still should check that that level is above MMin.)

Another approach is to estimate the air-conduction threshold, and use that when calculating the minimum masking level. If you calculate both the minimum and the maximum levels, then you can also choose any level between the two, with consideration of patient comfort.

If Using MinMask, Check for the Possibility of Overmasking

As you set the noise level in the non-test ear using a minimum masking level approach, always think "could this overmask?".

Take the noise level you are presenting. Subtract 45 dB (35 dB for supra-aural earphones), which is 5 dB less than the interaural attenuation value. Do you have concern that the bone-conduction threshold may be at or below that level? If so, you may be overmasking. Instead, use the maximum masking noise level approach or switch back to plateau masking.

Example

Child with a bilateral conductive loss, with flat tympanograms. Air-conduction thresholds in each ear are 50 dB HL.

Once I start masking, thresholds could increase, perhaps to 70 dB HL.

Minimum formula: *70 dB signal level – 40 dB + possible NTE 70 dB air-bone gap if the loss is as bad as 70 dB HL in each ear = 100 dB EM*

Maximum formula: *Best probable test ear bone-conduction threshold is 0 dB HL + 45 dB = 45.*

The maximum is 45, and the minimum is 100, obviously this is a problem! I will plateau mask and hope that the true interaural attenuation is higher than 70 (and lower than the amount of the conductive component). Maybe if I plateau carefully I will find a narrow, but present, plateau. Formula masking is not going to work. Even plateau masking may not work – this may be a masking dilemma.

Don't Formula Mask with Bilateral Conductive Losses

As the example above illustrates, if you have significant bilateral conductive loss, it's not safe to formula mask. You have to revert to plateau masking

Chapter 8 – Formula Masking – Air-Conduction

If Using MMax, Check that Masking is Sufficient

Some clinicians routinely use the MMax approach (with the level reduced to ensure that loudness discomfort isn't a problem.) If you use that strategy, do a final check that the masking was sufficient to mask the crossover. This is basically calculating the minimum masking level using the measured threshold:

Masked threshold – IA + 10 dB + NTE ABG. If you did not use at least this amount of noise, you are potentially undermasking.

Recognize the Need to Recalculate Masking Levels

You may need to recalculate the minimum masking level if you find the test ear air-conduction threshold is worse than you estimated or, when using MMax, if the test-ear bone conduction threshold was better than estimated.

When using a minimum masking level approach, you estimated the threshold. If you are finding that the patient's hearing threshold is above this level, pause. Recalculate your minimum masking level. Double check that this new level would not cause over masking. At this point, you either increase the masking noise and continue to search for threshold, or, if you found that you are at risk for overmasking, then stop the formula masking approach. Revert to plateau masking.

If you were using the MMax approach, then the concern is when bone-conduction thresholds for the test ear come in better than expected. You based the MMax on the bone-conduction threshold; if the patient's measured threshold is lower, then MMax is lower. In that case, re-consider potential for overmasking. (Simply recalculate MMax; if you used a noise above that level, retest the masked air-conduction threshold with a lower level of masking noise, one that is based on the new MMax or MMin.)

mQuest

The mQuest games, levels 10 and 11, ask you to calculate crossover, then establish the minimum masking level, which is simply 10 dB above the crossover for these levels, which involve sensorineural hearing loss. In level 10, the loss is unilateral; level 11 is very similar, the loss is bilateral but asymmetrical. Levels 10 and 11 also ask you for the maximum masking level: the test ear BC threshold + IA -5 dB (which simplifies to BC threshold + 45 for insert earphones). Remember that in the clinic, you can use any level between the minimum and maximum level and you will have masked appropriately

In Level 12, you first consider whether or not you should consider the possibility of air-bone gaps in the non-test ear. Look at the non-test ear immittance results. If they are normal, then assume that the bone-conduction threshold in the non-test ear equals the air-conduction threshold. If immittance is abnormal, assume that the bone-conduction threshold is 0 dB HL. If there are air-bone gaps in the non-test ear, you have to add the air-bone gaps to the NTE masking level. (The game is designed so that any air-bone gap cases will be significant air-bone gaps, not 5-10 dB ones that might leave you wondering what you should do.)

Remember that in formula masking, you have to estimate thresholds in order for your masking to be efficient. In level 10-12, you are given those estimated thresholds – that is what the "sliders" represent.

Chapter 8 – Formula Masking – Air-Conduction

Level 13 begins to have you estimate the test ear eventual threshold. You will be given one of the following scenarios:

- Prior testing indicates a "dead" ear. You would base your minimum masking formula on the audiometer's maximum output level (e.g. 125 dB HL).

- Prior testing gave you a given threshold level. Estimate that the threshold will be 20 dB worse – use that to calculate your minimum level. Your maximum should be based on the best possible bone-conduction threshold.

- You have a preliminary unmasked threshold at a given level. Guess that the eventual threshold will be 20 to 40 dB worse and use that to calculate your minimum masking level. Again, you'll calculate MMax.

Level 14 gives you the preliminary threshold, the twist is that there may be air-bone gaps in the test ear. In calculating your maximum masking level, you will need to use that best-possible bone-conduction threshold, which means that overmasking will be a problem more often.

Level 15 has possibilities of air-bone gaps both in the non-test ear and test ear. You will calculate crossover, the minimum and maximum masking values, and indicate if you should plateau mask instead. When you are getting absurd masking levels, (minimum is above maximum) remember – those are the times when, clinically, you would plateau

AudSim Flex

To move you towards mastery of air-conduction formula masking, it's time to use AudSim. You are not told to use a specific approach (min / max) – it's up to you to mask appropriately.

You can try some AudSim formula masking now, but until you have done bone-conduction formula masking, it's probably better to just try a few. I'd suggest doing more when you are ready to do both formula air- and bone-conduction masking.

With bilateral conductive loss, you can't safely formula mask – cases F, G, J, M, N, and P may require you revert to plateau masking, and you may have masking dilemmas. If you recognize that's the case, mark them as MD (masking dilemma) to indicate that you have recognized that you cannot plateau mask.

Chapter 8 – Formula Masking – Air-Conduction

Key Points

Any level between the minimum and maximum will mask appropriately; however, be considerate and avoid presenting uncomfortably loud masking levels.

- Formula masking works best if you estimate the final threshold accurately. If you estimate too low a threshold, you would need to readjust the masking levels upward.
- Sometimes, plateau masking is a better choice than formula masking. If you calculate MMin and MMax (using the same threshold in calculating both min and max) and they are the same or if MMax is lower than MMin, then you need to use plateau masking. (And if it is word discrimination testing or ABR testing, well, you are in a pickle. You'll have to do your best and note on the results the test limitation.) Chapter 10 discusses approaches to speech masking.

The formula are:

Minimum Masking Level (MMin):
TE signal level – IA + significant NTE ABG + 10 dB
 For insert earphones : TE signal level – 40 + NTE ABG
 For TDH headphones : TE signal level – 30 + NTE ABG
"Signal level" is your estimate of the eventual threshold, NOT the unmasked air-conduction threshold.

Maximum Masking Level (MMax):
BC threshold of the TE + IA – 5
 For insert earphones: TE best possible BC threshold - 45
 For TDH headphones: TE best possible BC threshold - 35

If you calculate both minimum and maximum and use a level within that range, you are sure to have masked correctly. If you use only the minimum masking formula, do a double check to be sure you are not overmasking :

Noise level – 45
If the TE BC threshold is that level or lower, you may be overmasking.

If you calculated only the maximum level, check to be sure you did not undermask. Once threshold is established, determine the signal level that crossed over. Could that be heard in the non-test ear, above the level of noise you used? (Alternatively, calculate MMin and be sure you used that much or more.)

Chapter 9

Formula Masking for Pure-Tone Bone-Conduction Testing

Quick Reference: The Formulae

Minimum Masking Level (Low Frequency)

In the low frequencies, where there is <u>an occlusion</u> effect:

Minimum Masking Level (MMin) =
Expected bone conduction threshold + 10 + (larger of: OE or NTE ABG)

Check for overmasking:
If Masking Level – 50 ≥ TE BC threshold, then overmasking may occur.

Minimum Masking Level (High Frequency)

In the high frequencies, where there is <u>no occlusion</u> effect:

Minimum Masking Level (MMin) =
Expected bone conduction threshold + 10 + any significant NTE ABG

Check for overmasking:
If Masking Level – 50 ≥ TE BC threshold, then overmasking may occur.

Maximum Masking Level (All Frequencies)

Maximum Masking Level (MMax) =
Lowest anticipated bone conduction threshold + 45 dB.

Check that masking is sufficient:
Calculate the Minimum Masking Level using the established BC threshold.
If MMin>MMax (based on the same estimate of the bone-conduction threshold), then plateau masking is needed.
Reminder: When in doubt, plateau it out.

When Testing Via Bone-Conduction, the Entire Stimulus Level Crosses Over to the NTE Cochlea

Before discussing the formula, this chapter first covers the theoretical foundation for building the formulae for the minimum and maximum masking levels. Let's start with considerations about crossover.

While there is some, though usually minimal, interaural attenuation for bone conduction, the audiology community's masking approach is to assume there is none. Whatever level bone-conduction stimulus is presented to the right ear crosses to the left cochlea (and of course, vice versa).

Chapter 9. Formula Masking – Bone Conduction

The air-conduction masking formula used "minus the interaural attenuation" value. Since bone conduction IA is assumed to be 0 dB, that won't be a part of the bone-conduction formula.

Occluding a Normal Non-Test Ear Enhances Bone-Conduction by Air-Conduction Signal Transmission, Increasing the Sound Level at the NTE Cochlea

Refer to Figure 9-1 below. It shows the process by which occluding the non-test ear with an insert earphone enhances the amount of sound that is sent via bone conduction, through the non-test ear's middle ear, to reach the cochlea.

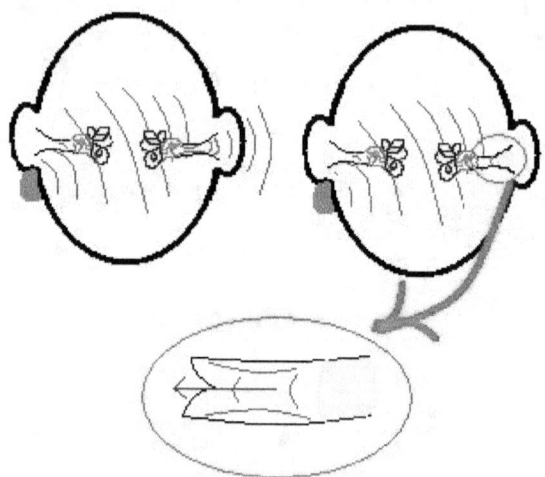

Figure 9-1. A. A bone oscillator on one mastoid vibrates the entire skull, including the bony portion of the contralateral external auditory canal. With the contralateral ear open, much of this air-conducted sound (created by the bone-conduction oscillator) escapes. (Left side of figure.) When the contralateral ear is occluded with an insert earphone, the sound does not escape. It is channeled into the middle ear and enhances the level of sound reaching the contralateral cochlea.

B. Another illustration of the same concept. The bone-conducted sound travels through the fused bones of the cranium to reach the non-test ear, which, when occluded by the earphone that will be used to present masking to the non-test ear, causes the sound coming from the vibration of the ear canals to be funneled into the middle ear, enhancing the sound that is present in the non-test ear cochlea. *(Figure B illustration credit: Heather Marinello)*

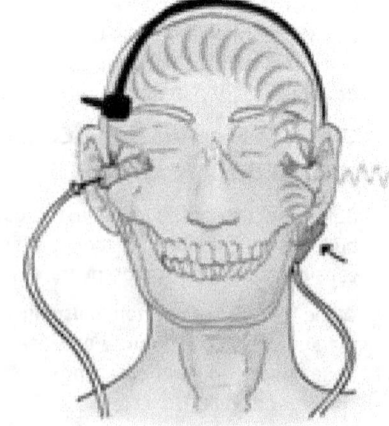

Recommended Occlusion Effect Values: 20/10/5/0 for Insert Earphones

Various studies estimate the occlusion effect (OE) values differently. This book recommends the following OE values. (If using TDH earphones, the OE values are a higher.)Chapter 6 contains the rationale for use of these values.

Table 9-1. Recommended occlusion effect (OE) values for insert earphones.

Frequency (Hz)	250	500	1k	Above 1k
OE Value	20	10	5	0

Table 9-2. Recommended occlusion effect (OE) values for TDH-style supra-aural earphones.

Frequency (Hz)	250	500	1k	Above 1k
OE Value	30	20	10	0

Increase the Masking Noise Intensity to Account for the Occlusion Effect

The level of the crossed-over bone-conduction signal, as enhancement from the occlusion effect, needs to be considered in the masking formula. If you are presenting a 40 dB, 500 Hz bone-conduction signal to the right ear, while occluding the left ear with an insert earphone so that you can mask, then the level of the signal reaching the left cochlea is 50 dB (add 10 for the occlusion effect). Your masking formula will need to account for the "boost" from the occlusion effect.

Conductive Loss in the Non-Test Ear Minimizes or Eliminates the Occlusion Effect

Assume that a normally hearing individual has a 20 dB occlusion effect at 250 Hz. If this patient develops a 5 dB conductive loss, then the occlusion effect is reduced to 15 dB. The conductive loss attenuates some of the sound level before it reaches the non-test ear cochlea. If the conductive loss is 20 dB or more, then no occlusion effect would be expected.

Depending upon the nature of the conductive loss, it is also possible that the patient already has an occlusion effect. An example would be cerumen occlusion of the non-test ear; it creates the occlusion effect, so the addition of the insert earphone doesn't add any additional effect.

Conductive Loss in the Non-Test Ear Reduces the Masking Level Reaching the NTE Cochlea

Chapter 9. Formula Masking – Bone Conduction

Masking is input to the non-test ear by air conduction; ergo, it will be reduced in intensity by any conductive hearing loss. Let's take the example of a non-test ear with 25 dB of conductive hearing loss. If you have crossover at 20 dB HL, and want 30 dB EM at the NTE cochlea (the 20 dB HL crossover plus an extra 10 dB "safety pad"), then you must input 55 dB of EM by air conduction. See Figure 9-2.

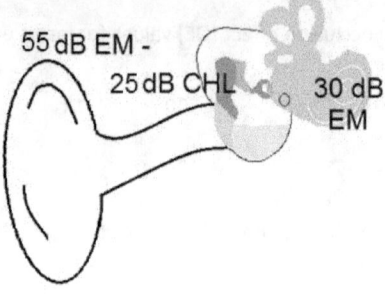

Figure 9-2. Conductive loss reduces the masking sound levels that reach the NTE cochlea. For example, 55 dB EM is attenuated by the 25 dB conductive hearing loss (CHL), so that only 30 dB EM reaches the non-test ear cochlea.

Include the Larger of the Occlusion Effect or Air-Bone Gap in Your Masking Formula, But Not Both

When the Occlusion Effect Value is Larger than the Air-Bone Gap at that Frequency, the Formula Uses the Occlusion Effect Value

Now let's examine the combined effect of the occlusion effect and conductive hearing loss. Assume we are presenting a 250 Hz, 30 dB HL bone-conducted sound to the test ear, and all of it crosses to the non-test ear. If the conductive loss is minor, for example, 10 dB at 250 Hz, the occlusion effect would enhance the 30 dB of crossover by 20 dB, but the conductive loss would reduce the amount of the occlusion effect that reaches the NTE cochlea (by 10 dB in this example). The net (+ occlusion effect – conductive loss) is 10 dB in this example of minor conductive involvement. The bone-conducted sound is enhanced, but only by 10 dB.

The masking noise has to be channeled into this ear with the conductive component; therefore, the masking noise needs to be increased 10 dB to compensate for the conductive loss. So, above we subtracted out the conductive component in order to determine the adjusted size of the occlusion effect. Now, in this next step, we are adding in the size of the conductive hearing loss to ensure that we have enough masking level reaching the non-test ear cochlea. The masking adjustment = Occlusion Effect – Air-Bone Gap Size + Air-Bone Gap Size. That zeros out the conductive component size (the air-bone gap size) in the masking equation. So, when the conductive component is smaller than the occlusion effect, you can just ignore it.

One more time? When you have a case of minor conductive loss in the non-test ear, adjust the masking level by adding the remaining occlusion effect (OE – conductive loss size) plus the conductive loss size to compensate for the eventual loss due to the masking noise having to go through the outer and middle ear. The math simplifies to: add the OE.

In the example discussed above, where the occlusion effect is larger than the conductive loss size,
e.g. (20 dB OE – 10 cond loss) + 10 cond loss = 20,
you can ignore the conductive loss size and just add in the occlusion effect.

To summarize:
If the occlusion effect size is larger than the air-bone gap size, the formula does not need to be adjusted. Just use the occlusion effect value.

When the Air-Bone Gap is Larger than the Occlusion Effect Value at that Frequency, the Formula Uses the NTE Air-Bone Gap Size

There is no "negative" occlusion effect: it can only be reduced to zero. A negative occlusion effect number would mean that the middle ear pathology is reducing the crossover. Obviously, that makes no sense – the middle ear condition isn't going to stop the bone-conduction crossover! So, in cases where the conductive loss is larger than the occlusion effect, the occlusion effect becomes zero.

The adjustment needed to the masking level is as follows:

(No occlusion effect) + conductive loss size.

We need to compensate for the fact that the masking noise will be reduced by the conductive loss. Remember that the crossover goes to the non-test ear cochlea, so we need to have enough masking noise reach the cochlea. We have to increase the air-conducted masking noise intensity by the amount of the NTE conductive loss to have the desired level reach the cochlea.

To summarize:
If the air-bone gap is larger than the occlusion effect size, adjust the masking formula:
Add the air-bone gap size, but not the occlusion effect size.

Summary of the Bone-Conduction Formula Principles

Conductive hearing loss in the non-test ear complicates bone-conduction masking.

In the **low frequencies**, where there is an occlusion effect, **increase the masking noise by the larger of the size of the occlusion effect OR the size of the air-bone gap in the non-test ear.**
Use one or the other, not both.

In the **high frequencies**, where there is no occlusion effect, **adjust the noise to compensate for the conductive loss magnitude.**

How to Determine the NTE Conductive Loss Size; Complications from Air-Bone Gaps in the NTE

Especially if you work with adults, the hearing loss tends to most often be sensorineural. In those cases where there is conductive loss in the non-test ear the masking has to be adjusted. In "which came first the chicken or the egg" fashion, we have to add in the non-test ear air-bone gap size before we have conducted masked bone-conduction testing on that ear. All is not lost, we will see how we can make an estimate that may allow formula masking.

Chapter 9. Formula Masking – Bone Conduction

Reminder – with Bilateral Conductive Loss Plateau Masking is Preferrable, Partially Because You Don't Know the NTE Air-Bone Gap Size

Typically the audiologist will conduct unmasked bone-conduction testing on the better ear first. If you discover air-bone gaps, then . . . well, if the loss may be conductive bilaterally, then you may be running into a really challenging masking case, and potentially a masking dilemma, so you might want to plateau mask the better ear first.

Sometimes You May Not Need to Mask Bone-Conduction for the Better Ear

Joke: Did you know that Spock (of Space Ship Enterprise fame) had three ears? His left ear, his right ear, and the final front ear. But I digress.

You might also decide to leave the better ear bone-conduction thresholds unmasked for the time being. You could plateau mask the better ear later. If the poorer ear's hearing is significantly worse (e.g. sensorineural loss), you may not need to mask that better ear at all. The "bad" ear threshold is elevated beyond what the unmasked threshold showed. If you are sure of your masking results, then the unmasked scores must be for the better ear's cochlea, (unless your patient is Spock and has a third ear.)

Example of When to Add the NTE Air-Bone Gaps to the Masking Formula

If you think the conductive loss is only in the better ear, you can formula mask when you test the poorer ear – add in the larger of either the occlusion effect or the air-bone gap size. So, let's explore that case further, referencing Figure 9-3. As you start testing the right ear (poorer ear) by bone conduction, make the assumption that the left ear (better hearing ear) loss is conductive. (If you already plateau masked, you know exactly the size of the conductive loss.)

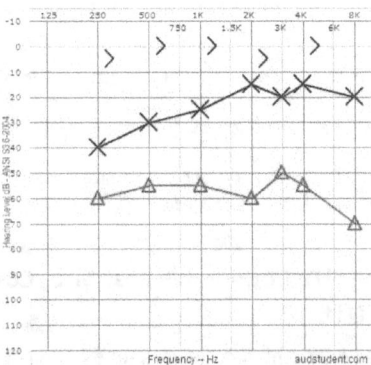

Figure 9-3. When calculating the needed masking in order to test right bone-conduction hearing, assume that the unmasked left ear bone-conduction scores truly reflect the cochlear sensitivity of the left ear, and use those air-bone gap sizes. Above, the air-bone gaps are larger than the occlusion effect values, so the occlusion effect is omitted from the masking formula; the air-bone gap size is added. At 2000 Hz the air-bone gap size is small, but it still should be added to the masking formula. It is likely a "real" air-bone gap.

Options for Dealing with Minor Air-Bone Gaps

Remember: if the air-bone gaps are smaller than, or equal to, the size of the occlusion effect, just add the occlusion effect value (Figure 9-4 left.) If there are only minor air-bone gaps, which appear to be the result of test/retest variability (Figure 9-4 right), then including that air-bone gap in the masking formula is optional. The most cautious approach is to add in air-bone gaps if you are not sure if they are or are not truly reflecting conductive involvement; so, if there is any doubt, include the air-bone gap.

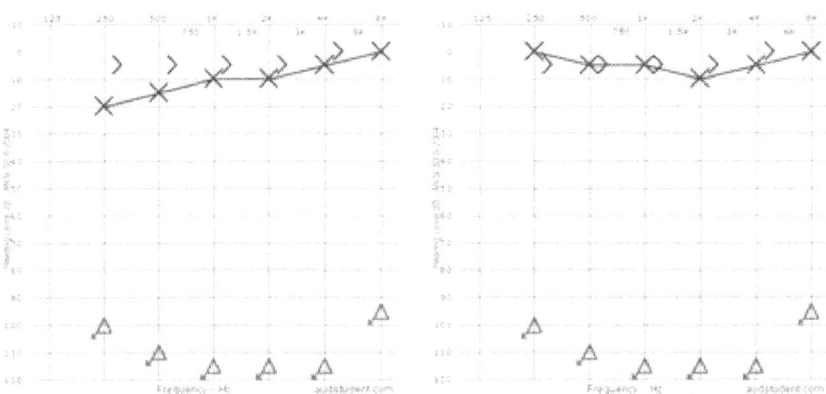

Figure 9-4. Left side of figure. There is a pattern of air-bone gaps in the low frequencies, and they appear to indicate conductive involvement. When calculating the masking noise needed, one would add in the occlusion effect values (20 dB at 250, 10 dB at 500 Hz, 5 dB at 1000 Hz), because those values are equal to or larger than the air-bone gap. At 2000 and 4000 Hz, it would be appropriate to add the air-bone gaps to the formula. Although the air-bone gaps are small, they appear to be "real" – it is likely that the masking noise will be attenuated 5 dB as it passes through the middle ear. Right side of figure. In this case, and especially so if patient symptoms and/or immittance testing are indicating that there is not a conductive component to the loss, adding the air-bone gaps is not necessary. They are not "real" air-bone gaps – they reflect test/re-test variability in thresholds. However, it does not usually hurt to add in these minor air-bone gaps. Ignore any bone-air gaps (e.g. 250 Hz).

Importance of the 10 dB "Safety Pad" in Bone-Conduction Formula Masking

With air-conduction testing we have two "safety nets" to help keep us from undermasking. We add the 10 dB in our formula as a "safety pad", and we assume a 50 dB interaural attenuation (for insert earphones.) In reality, interaural attenuation is likely to be much higher. With bone-conduction masking you don't have that interaural attenuation portion of the safety net, so if there is any question about the air-bone gap being real, add it to your minimum masking level calculation. Ensure that you always have at least the 10 dB extra masking in case the patient's occlusion effect values are larger than average, or if there is a minor calibration error in your masking output levels.

Chapter 9. Formula Masking – Bone Conduction

Part One of Self-Check on Handling NTE Air-Bone Gaps

What is the masking formula adjustment that you should use if there are large air-bone gaps in the non-test ear, that is, larger than the occlusion effect size?

Increase the masking amount by adding:

    a) The air-bone gap size only

    b) The occlusion effect size only

    c) Both the air-bone gap and occlusion effect size

a. Add in only the air-bone gap. The occlusion effect has been eliminated – the additional "bone-conduction by air-conduction" sound is attenuated to 0 dB as it goes through the conductive loss in the non-test ear.

Part Two of Self-Check on Handling NTE Air-Bone Gaps

What is the masking formula adjustment that you should use when testing 1000 Hz and below, if there are small air-bone gaps in the non-test ear; that is, they probably are real, but they are smaller than the occlusion effect size?

Increase the masking amount by adding:

    a) The air-bone gap size only

    b) The occlusion effect size only

    c) Both the air-bone gap and occlusion effect size

b. Add in the occlusion effect, ignore the air-bone gaps. Even if they are real (not just test-retest variability), they don't matter. If you were to make an adjustment, step one would be to reduce masking by the size of the conductive loss, and step two would be to increase the masking by the size of the occlusion effect. That cancels out the minor conductive loss's effect, so you can just ignore small air-bone gaps.

Part Three of Self-Check on Handling NTE Air-Bone Gaps

What is the masking formula adjustment that you should use when testing the high frequencies, where there is no occlusion effect, if there are small air-bone gaps in the non-test ear?

Assume that you have reason to believe these are real air-bone gaps (e.g. the ear has abnormal immittance results).

    a) Increase the masking amount by adding in the air-bone gap size

    b) Ignore the air-bone gap

Chapter 9. Formula Masking – Bone Conduction

a. Increase the masking level. You don't have much of a "safety cushion" in bone-conduction masking. If the noise is going to be reduced by a conductive loss, then you need to increase the masking noise to compensate.

Vibrotactile Bone-Conduction Thresholds

Defined

If thresholds are sufficiently elevated, the responses measured may be responses to feeling the sound vibration rather than hearing the sound: they are potentially vibrotactile responses. Thresholds at or above those noted in Table 9-3 potentially may be vibrotactile.

Table 9-3. Lowest levels at which a vibrotactile response would be expected.

Frequency (Hz)	250	500	1000
Air Conduction (dB HL)	85	105	120
Bone Conduction (dB HL)	25	55	75

If BC Thresholds May Be Vibrotactile, but Conductive Involvement is Possible, then Add the Apparent Air-Bone Gaps to the Minimal Masking Formula

If the patient has bone-conduction thresholds that may be vibrotactile, then what appears on the audiogram as a mixed loss may in reality be a sensorineural loss. If there is doubt – maybe the responses are hearing and maybe there is a conductive component to the loss – then treat the potentially vibrotactile thresholds as if they are hearing thresholds. Include any resulting air-bone gaps in the masking formulae.

When You Find Vibrotactile Bone-Conduction Thresholds, Omit Apparent Air-Bone Gaps if Conductive Involvement is Not Suspected

If you are sure the responses are vibrotactile (e.g. the patient tells you that s/he felt the sound rather than hearing it; immittance testing is consistent with normal middle ear function), then the apparent air-bone gaps are of no concern. You do not need to add them to your masking formula. I would recommend marking the bone-conduction thresholds as "VT" for "vibrotactile". (Pen in the VT notation next to the bone-conduction symbol on the audiogram. Make a comment if using a computer-based audiometer.) Vibrotactile responses will not shift with contralateral masking, so if you do mask, and the thresholds do shift, then they were not vibrotactile. (I can make an argument for a small central masking effect; the patient may be distracted from the threshold level vibration sensation by contralateral noise, but in general, thresholds of feeling aren't going to be altered by contralateral masking.)

Chapter 9. Formula Masking – Bone Conduction

Overmasking

Bone-Conduction Over Masking Calculations Use the Air-Conduction Interaural Attenuation Value

The concerns about overmasking are the same as for air-conduction testing. The air-conducted NOISE presented to the NON-test ear can become BONE-conducted sound that crosses BACK to the TEST ear COCHLEA. To estimate the amount of noise that could cross back, subtract 50 dB (the estimated interaural air-conduction attenuation value for insert earphones) from the masking noise level being used.

If the test ear bone-conduction threshold you are measuring is at or below (smaller number than) the crossback level, then the bone-conduction threshold is potentially elevated by the overmasking. Said differently, the reason you are measuring as high a bone-conduction threshold as you are could be because the noise crossed back to the test ear cochlea and that masking level prevented hearing of threshold level sounds. The test ear threshold is artificially made poorer because of overmasking.

A Graphical Approach to Thinking About Masking for Bone Conduction

Asymmetrical Sensorineural Loss

It is common to need to mask bone conduction for a unilateral sensorineural loss case, so let's begin with that case. Read the figure legends as you go along.

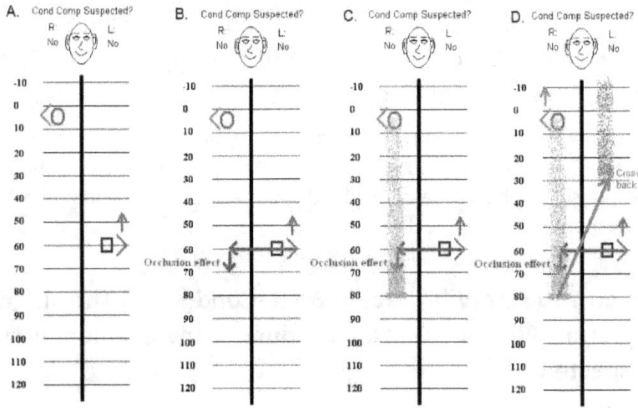

Figure 9-5. 500 Hz testing (10 dB occlusion effect). A. Assume that the right ear hearing is normal. The threshold was 5 dB HL both by air- and bone-conduction. If you do not think the left ear loss is conductive, then your guess is that the bone-conduction threshold will be 60 dB HL. Of course, it may be better than that, as suggested by the arrow.

B. Since there is no interaural attenuation for bone conduction, the crossover is 60 dB HL. The test frequency is 500 Hz; there is an expectation of a 10 dB occlusion effect. The level at the right ear cochlea is 70 dB HL

C. Putting in 80 dB EM into the right ear should mask the crossover. You should give a little cushion in case the patient's occlusion effect is higher than 10 dB, or in case there is a small masking noise calibration error.

Chapter 9. Formula Masking – Bone Conduction

D. Assuming a 50 dB IA, the level of noise that could cross back is 30 dB HL. If the test ear bone-conduction threshold is 30 dB or better (e.g. 25 dB HL), then overmasking may be shifting the left ear bone-conduction threshold. You may be overmasking. If the loss is, as expected, sensorineural, then the presence of the 30 dB EM crossback won't affect hearing of the 60 dB HL bone-conduction pure tone in the left ear.

Summary: Minimum Masking Level for Bone-Conduction Crossover and Cross Back with Bilateral Sensorineural Loss

MMin = TE BC signal level + 10 dB + Larger of OE or NTE ABG.
Crossback check: Noise – 50. OK unless measured BC threshold is this or lower.

As the discussion above has indicated, if you present a certain level bone-conduction signal, assume all the sound has crossed over. To ensure sufficient masking noise, you add in the larger of the occlusion effect size or the air-bone gap size. Add 10 more dB. That is enough to mask that crossover.

Crossback is calculated by taking the (air-conduction) noise level and subtracting 50 dB, the "worst-case" interaural attenuation value for insert earphones. If the test ear's bone-conduction hearing is at that value or has better hearing (lower dB number threshold) then there is concern that overmasking has occurred.

Game Time: mQuest Level 16

If you are having trouble keeping all the ideas straight, well, you're normal. And even if this makes perfect sense to you, it's still a good idea to cement the concepts using some game practice. Play game level 16 in mQuest. It will give you practice at examining crossover, and thinking about how it was enhanced by the occlusion effect. The game also asks you to find the crossback level. Level 16 includes unilateral and asymmetrical sensorineural hearing loss cases.

Air-Bone Gaps Complicate Formula Masking

In order for formula masking to be more time efficient than plateau masking, you have to make good estimates of the thresholds you expect to eventually measure. When immittance is abnormal in either the test or non-test ear, this complicates considerations of what masking is enough, and what will be too much.

If You Expected SNHL and the TE Loss is Actually Mixed or Conductive, Overmasking May Be a Problem

Remember that overmasking happens when the crossback level is at or higher than the test ear bone-conduction threshold.

While formula masking, you need to make an estimate of the expected test-ear bone-conduction threshold. If you expected that the loss will be sensorineural, then use the air-conduction threshold as the estimate of the expected bone-conduction threshold. If, when establishing the threshold, you find the bone-conduction threshold comes in better than expected (the test ear loss is mixed or conductive), then you may need to re-adjust the masking level to a lower intensity to avoid overmasking. Figure 9-6 illustrates.

Chapter 9. Formula Masking – Bone Conduction

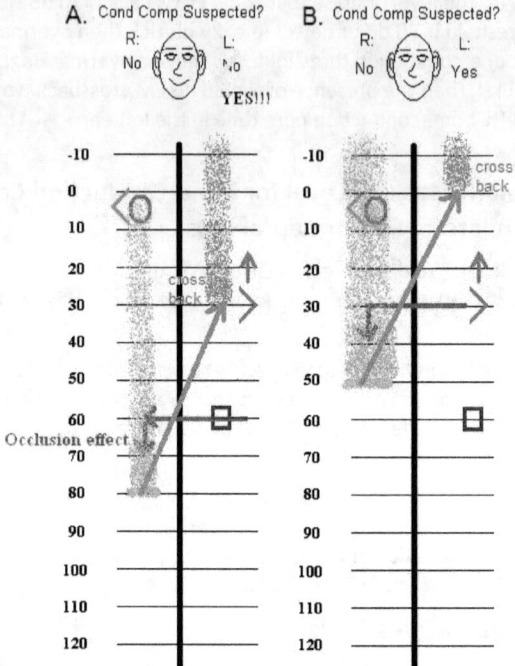

Figure 9-6. Example of 500 Hz testing (10 dB occlusion effect).

A. SNHL was expected. Masking level used = signal level (estimated threshold of 60 dB) + 10 dB OE + 10 dB pad = 80 dB EM. If you find that the bone-conduction threshold is better than expected, and may be elevated by the crossback, then you have based your formula on too high an estimated bone-conduction threshold.

B. Recalculate the minimum masking level based on the lowered estimate of the bone-conduction threshold. (30 dB expected BC threshold + 10 dB OE + 10 dB pad = 50 dB EM.) Now the cross-back (0 dB EM) is not going to affect your test results unless the bone-conduction threshold comes in at 0 dB HL or better, in which case you can reduce the masking noise further. (That's unlikely since the unmasked bone-conduction threshold is 5 dB HL.)

Next mQuest Game Level 17

In mQuest level 17, you will play out the following scenario. Without the benefit of immittance test results for the test ear, you initially assume that the test ear loss is sensorineural and calculate the crossover and minimum masking levels, and then evaluate the potential crossback level. The measured threshold is then given to you, and often the loss is not what you expected: The test ear has conductive or mixed loss. You will determine if it could be elevated due to overmasking: is the NTE masking is crossing back? If so, you will reduce the masking level as needed.

Chapter 9. Formula Masking – Bone Conduction

Large NTE Air-Bone Gaps: Add the Air-Bone Gap to the Masking Level (Not the OE)

As already discussed, if conductive loss (larger than the OE size) is present in the non-test ear, then the NTE masking intensity needs to be increased to compensate, so that the desired level reaches the NTE cochlea. Read Figure 9-7 legends.

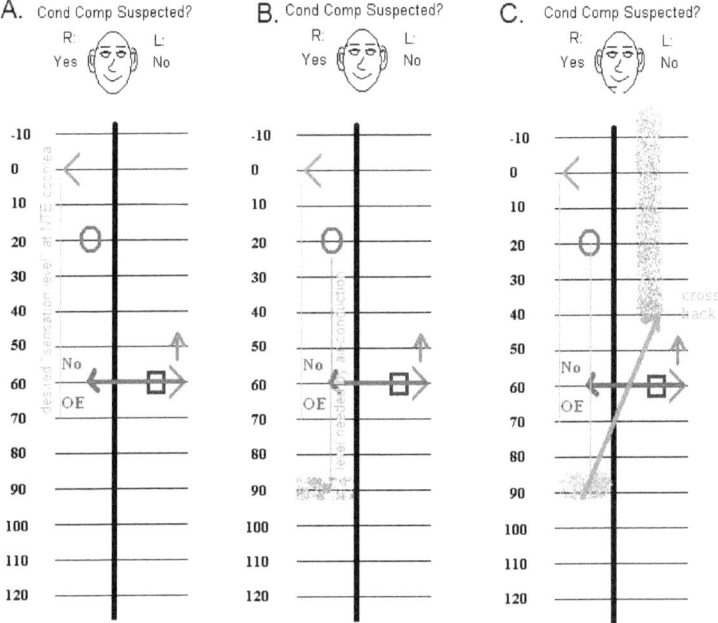

Figure 9-7. Regardless of which frequency is being tested, an occlusion effect value is NOT needed since the right ear (NTE) air-bone gap is equal to or larger than the largest occlusion effect value (assuming you are testing with insert earphones)

A. The goal is to have 70 dB more effective masking than the NTE bone-conduction threshold (60 dB crossover + 10 dB pad).

B. Because there is conductive loss in the non-test ear, increase the masking noise by the amount of that NTE air-bone gap. This keeps the noise at the desired level when it reaches the NTE cochlea.

C. Overmasking could be a problem if the test ear bone-conduction threshold is 40 dB HL or if testing reveals even less impairment.

Bilateral Mixed or Conductive Hearing Loss: You May Want To, or Need To, Plateau Mask

Conductive loss in the non-test ear increases the masking level needed. If the test ear bone-conduction threshold is relatively normal, this creates a situation where overmasking is likely, in which case one would plateau mask, if that is possible. In Figure 9-8 A, the noise level was too high, but because the bone-conduction value in the test ear was better than anticipated, the masking noise can be reduced (part B of the figure). Formula masking is still possible. Part C of the figure shows the case where the NTE ABG is large, and equal to the expected test ear ABG. In this case, formula masking is impossible. You know that you may be overmasking as soon as you begin testing.

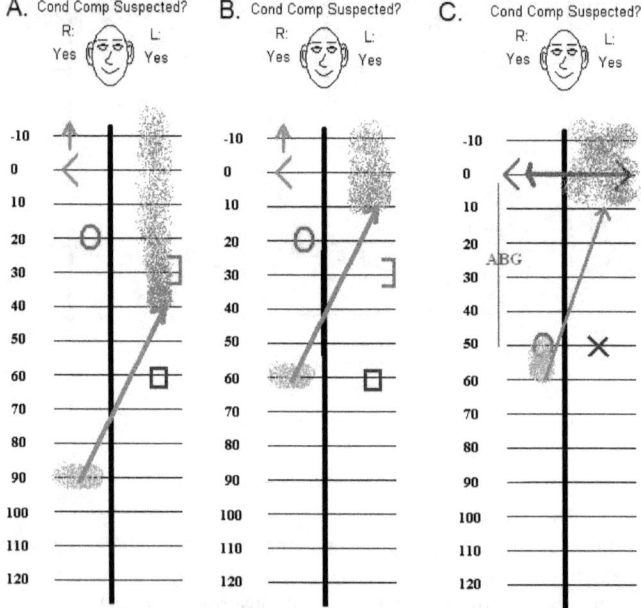

Figure 9-8. 500 Hz testing with bilateral mixed/conductive loss. The non-test ear is assumed to have normal cochlear sensitivity.

A. The masking level was calculated assuming the loss would be sensorineural in the left ear. (60 dB expected bone-conduction threshold + 20 dB NTE ABG + 10 dB = 90 dB EM). In reality, a 30 dB HL threshold was measured. Overmasking is problematic: the crossback (90-50) may be 40 dB EM. Because the measured threshold is lower than 40dB crossback, the masking noise intensity must be decreased.

B. Recalculating the masking noise needed may allow formula masking. (30 dB or better bone-conduction threshold + 20 dB NTE ABG + 10 = 60 dB EM). Here, crossback could be 10 dB EM. If you find the threshold is 10 dB HL or lower, you need to reduce the noise level yet again. If you are continually having to adjust your noise levels, it may be safer and easier to plateau mask.

Chapter 9. Formula Masking – Bone Conduction

C. When the air-bone gaps in each ear are large, then we cannot safely formula mask. When we assume that the interaural attenuation value for the air-conducted masking noise is 50 dB, we can recognize that we have the potential for overmasking. Plateau masking is needed. (Expected TE BC threshold of 0 dB crosses over + 50 dB NTE air-bone gap + 10 dB = 60. Crossback (60-50= 10 dB EM) is 10 dB EM, which is above the expected test ear bone-conduction threshold.

Deeply Insert the Insert Earphones to Minimize the Crossback

Remember, air-conduction interaural attenuation values are generally higher than 50 dB, so plateau masking may work when formula masking does not. Deeply inserting the insert earphone that is delivering the masking noise reduces the amount of ear canal surface area that vibrates, and this means it creates less of an occlusion effect and the interaural attenuation is greater (Figure 9-9). A larger interaural attenuation value means ther will be less crossback.

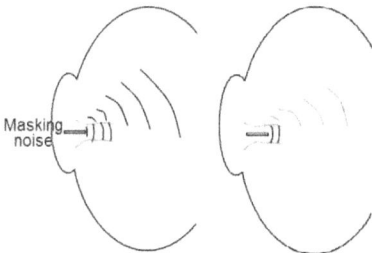

Figure 9-9. Masking noise crossback is minimized by use of a deeply inserted insert earphone because less surface area of the ear canal is vibrating. Additionally, a deeply inserted earphone reduces the occlusion effect size.

Step-by-Step Approach to the Bone-Conduction Minimum Masking Level Calculations

Next we apply the concepts covered and go through the complete sequence of steps in the minimal masking level approach.

Step one. Estimate the bone-conduction threshold of the test ear.

To be efficient, to minimize the number of times that you have to adjust the masking level, it helps to have a good guess of the test ear bone-conduction threshold, which is the first step in the Minimum Masking Level Formula. If you have prior test results, those can guide you; otherwise, here are two ways to estimate the test ear bone-conduction threshold.

Option A. If predicting normal TE BC hearing, estimate a 20 to 30 dB HL BC threshold

If you believe that the test ear loss is conductive, you are assuming that the bone-conduction threshold will be 0 dB HL. But to be efficient you don't want to set the masking based only on that guess, because if the threshold comes in a bit higher than 0 dB HL, you

Chapter 9. Formula Masking – Bone Conduction

will have to increase the noise level. If you think that the bone conduction scores will be normal, base your minimum level calculations on a threshold such as 20 or 30 dB HL. If you have an unmasked threshold, base your minimum masking formula on a threshold 20-30 dB higher than that level.

Option B. Use the unmasked BC threshold as your estimate, adding 20 to 30 dB to reduce risk of undermasking

If you have already tested unmasked bone-conduction on the better ear, the test ear masked threshold won't be better than that. Again, to reduce the number of times you need to adjust, make the calculation of the minimum masking level needed with the assumption that the test ear will have a 20 to 30 dB higher bone-conduction threshold.

Option C. If predicting SNHL, use TE AC threshold or maximum output level

If you believe the test ear loss is sensorineural, then use the air-conduction threshold as your estimate of the bone-conduction threshold. However, if bone-conduction testing cannot be completed at that high an intensity (e.g. a 90 dB HL air-conduction threshold and a 70 dB HL bone-conduction maximum output limit on the audiometer), then you don't need to estimate a threshold higher than what the audiometer would produce. Use the maximum output limit for bone conduction, at that frequency, when estimating the threshold – which in this case is the level at which you expect to mark "no response".

Step two. Add the larger of the occlusion effect size or the NTE conductive hearing loss size

In the high frequencies, there is no occlusion effect, so just add in the conductive loss size. Remember: the safest action is to include even small air-bone gaps unless you have good reason to believe the air-bone gap is just the result of test/retest variability. At 1k Hz and below where there is an occlusion effect, add whichever is larger: the OE size or the ABG size.

Step three. Add a 10 dB "safety pad"

This step is critical – we must be sure we have enough masking in case the occlusion effect is larger than expected.

Step four. Apply this level noise to the non-test ear and establish/confirm TE hearing threshold

If you recognized the need to mask, and haven't bothered to get an unmasked threshold for this ear, good for you! You have saved time, and your patient will appreciate your efficiency. Just obtain the masked threshold, adjusting the test ear level using the Hughson-Westlake approach.

If you have already established the unmasked bone-conduction threshold, present again at this level. If the tone is still heard, then mark the masked threshold. If the threshold is higher than the unmasked bone-conduction threshold, then use the standard Hughson-Westlake method to find the masked bone-conduction threshold.

Step five. Consider potential undermasking. Undermasking is not a concern if the measured threshold is at or lower than the value you estimated. If the BC threshold is higher than expected, undermasking may be occurring. Recalculate minimum masking levels and retest.

After finding the masked bone-conduction threshold, check -- did you estimate the bone conduction threshold correctly?

If the threshold you found on your patient is at or lower than what you guessed, that is, you over-estimated the loss severity or estimated correctly, then your masking is sufficient: You have not undermasked. Mark the threshold, turn off your masking noise. Go on to the next step.

If you guessed wrong, and the threshold is higher than anticipated (e.g. you guessed a 50 dB HL threshold and the measured threshold is 60 dB HL), then you will need to make another estimate of the final bone-conduction threshold, and recalculate the masking noise that is needed based on this new guess. (Turn up the noise level.) In making the next estimate of threshold, go higher than what you have just measured – usually by 20 dB or more. The reason for increasing your guess of the test ear bone-conduction threshold by at least 20 dB is that if your estimated threshold (upon which you recalculate the masking noise) is only marginally higher than your original estimate, you are more likely to be wrong again, and have to yet again turn up the noise. If you are calculating and re-upping the masking noise continually, that is no more efficient than plateau masking.

Step six. Check for overmasking: Determine if overmasking may have made your results invalid. If you have overmasked, recalculate the noise level and re-establish threshold. If you did not overmask, then you can proceed to test the next frequency

To check for overmasking, note the noise level that you used. Subtract 50 dB – the minimum interaural attenuation value for insert earphones. If the bone-conduction threshold you just measured is at that level or lower (less impairment), then your results may have been influenced by overmasking. The noise may have crossed back to the test cochlea and masked the test ear signal. You will need to lower the noise level.

If you are potentially overmasking, and if the masking noise level was based on an estimate of the bone-conduction threshold that turned out to be too high (e.g. you guessed a 50 dB HL threshold, and you measured a 30 dB HL threshold), then recalculate the masking noise needed based on this lower threshold: try again.

If instead, the guess was pretty accurate, but you still are calculating that overmasking may be problematic, then it is likely you can't formula mask. You will need to use a plateau masking approach in order to be confident of your test results.

Back to mQuest – Level 18

Level 18 steps you through the minimum masking approach. You'll be given the non-test ear air- and bone-conduction thresholds and test ear air-conduction threshold. You will be asked to estimate the test ear bone-conduction threshold, and then determine the minimum masking level required. In some instances, the game will then tell you the

Chapter 9. Formula Masking – Bone Conduction

measured test ear bone-conduction threshold, and you'll be asked if that may be overmasking. If so, you'll calculate a new minimum masking level.

Concepts Related to Using the Maximum Masking Formula (MMax): Lowest anticipated bone conduction threshold + 45 dB

The approach described above involves predicting threshold, and using that as the basis for setting the minimum masking level. Using that minimum level allows the patient to be exposed to the lowest possible noise levels. The alternative approach – finding the maximum masking level – involves using as much noise as possible without risking overmasking. To use this approach, you consider the lowest (reasonably) possible TE bone-conduction threshold and base the masking noise on a level that will not overmask.

Strategies for Selecting the Lowest Anticipated TE BC Threshold

If you suspect conductive or mixed loss in the TE:

- Base your MMax value on an estimate of a -10 to 0 dB HL threshold or
- If you have a prior audiogram on the patient, and have no reason to think hearing has improved, then estimate that you will find the BC threshold as 10 dB better than the last test. By selecting a value a little lower, you won't have to adjust the masking level if, due to test/retest variability, the BC threshold is slightly better.
- If you believe the loss is sensorineural, it's still best to guess that the threshold will come in 10 to 20 dB lower than the AC threshold. If there are minor, insignificant air-bone gaps, having based your masking formula on the lower threshold keeps you from having to lower your masking level.

With severe and profound sensorineural loss, the AC thresholds may be above the maximum bone-conduction output limits. MMax is still based on cochlear sensitivity – you can base MMax on that value rather than the maximum output of the audiometer. This will give you a very high MMax – higher than you will want to use. Currently level 19 in mQuest is going to knock you down to the maximum audiometer output level. I might change that in the future, but it's really not important. Adding 45 dB to the air-conduction threshold or to the maximum output of the audiometer gives you a very high MMax! Remember, clinically, don't use a level at MMax if that will cause loudness discomfort.

Chapter 9. Formula Masking – Bone Conduction

Once You Estimate Lowest Anticipated TE BC Threshold, Add 45 dB: That is MMax

To obtain MMax, add 45 dB to the anticipated bone-conduction threshold -- don't use a masking noise level higher than this. Why 45? The interaural attenuation for air-conduction masking is 50 dB. We can safely use up to 45 dB more noise than the test ear bone-conduction threshold without concern that the crossback will interfere with the patient's hearing of the test ear tone. As long as your established (measured) bone-conduction threshold is NOT LOWER than what you estimated as the bone-conduction threshold when making the maximum level calculation, then you will not have risked overmasking.

To recap:
The maximum noise formula (MMax) is:
Lowest anticipated bone-conduction threshold + 45 dB.

MMax Approach Requires Checking for Undermasking

Using the maximum masking level approach guards against overmasking (assuming your estimated bone-conduction threshold was low enough), but it doesn't ensure that you are not undermasking. Therefore, you need to ensure that the masking noise was sufficient. Calculate the minimum masking level.

Checking for Undermasking with Minimal or No NTE Air-Bone Gaps: Calculate the Minimum Using the OE Values

If the occlusion effect is larger than the NTE ABG (or there is no ABG), then we must take into account the added intensity that the crossover takes on due to the non-test ear occlusion effect enhancing the "bone-conduction by air-conduction" hearing mechanism.

If OE is larger than NTE ABG, you are not undermasking if:

TE BC threshold + OE + 10 dB ≤ Masking noise level (MMax).

You want at least the 10 dB "safety pad", so MMax must be at or above this calculated MMin, which includes that 10 dB safety pad. The 10 dB pad is important because some people will have occlusion effects larger than the 20/10/5 dB estimates (at 250/500/1000 Hz respectively).

Checking for Undermasking with Large NTE Air-Bone Gaps: Adjust the Minimum Masking Formula Accordingly

To double check that your masking level was sufficient, **if the NTE ABG is larger than the occlusion effect** value for that frequency, then use the air-bone gap size in the minimum masking calculation. Stated as a formula:

If NTE has ABG larger than OE, you are not undermasking if:

TE BC threshold + NTE ABG + 10 dB ≤ Masking noise level (MMax).

Even though you are not concerned about a larger than average occlusion effect when there are large NTE air-bon gaps, you still want the 10 dB safety pad. If your masking noise calibration is slightly off, or if the true air-bone gap is a bit larger, it is helpful to have this extra "cushion". If you don't have that extra 10 dB of masking that is built into the MMin formula, you risk undermasking.

Check for Sufficient Masking After Finding Threshold

The astute reader notices that, when using the MMax approach, you aren't avoiding calculating the minimum masking level, so one may ask, why not do both calculations from the start? You could, and in cases of sensorineural loss that works well – choose a masking level between MMin and MMax. However, it's easier to do the check afterwards. When you calculated MMax, you thought about the best possible bone-conduction threshold. When we were calculating the minimum level, we were estimating a bit higher bone-conduction threshold so that we didn't have to readjust the masking levels. Rather than guessing the final level, the check of whether you used enough masking becomes more straight forward if you use the bone-conduction threshold that you established while using the MMax level.

What To Do If MMax was Insufficient Masking

If you calculated Mmax, and now find that you don't have enough masking noise, one of two things is happening. You may have bilateral conductive loss and a potential masking dilemma. In that case, plateau mask. Another reason for undermasking is that your estimate of the test ear bone-conduction threshold was lower than the actual measured threshold. (You guessed a low threshold, the real threshold was worse than that.) In that case, your new mMax is higher. You probably can increase the masking noise intensity level.

Examples

Figure 9-10 shows an example where the NTE has an air-bone gap larger than the occlusion effect value.

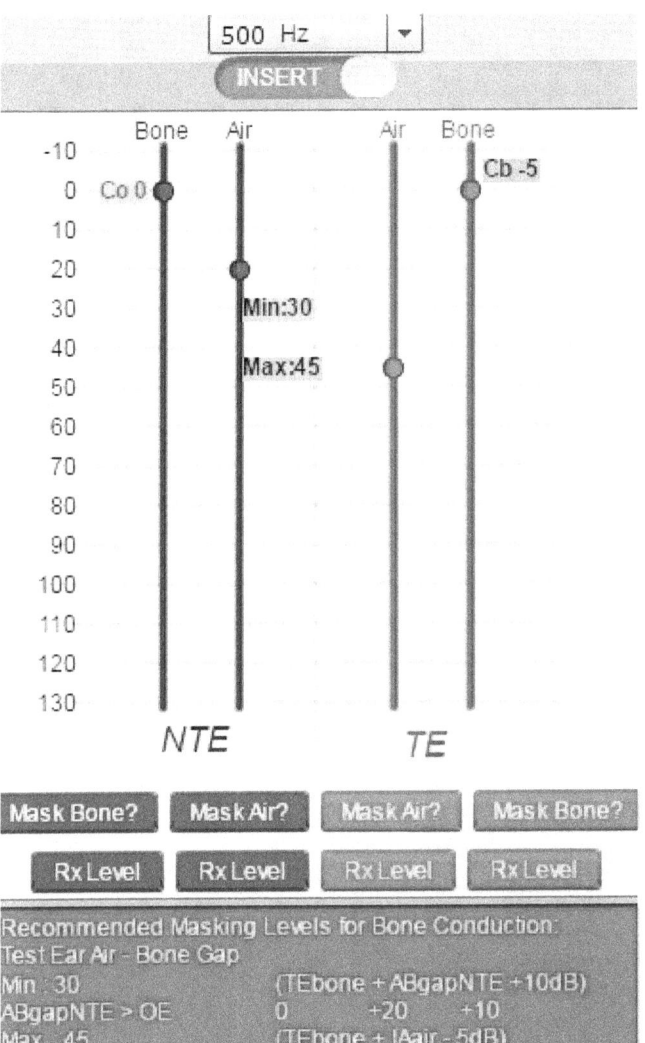

Figure 9-10. It was assumed that there could be conductive loss in the test ear, so the conservative estimate of a test ear threshold of 0 dB was chosen. The MMax is 0 + 45. Let's examine the case where a 0 dB threshold is found, as was expected. The next step is to check that the masking was sufficient. 0 dB BC threshold + 20 dB NTE ABG + 10 =30. The minimum needed level is 30 dB HL, MMax is higher. Masking was sufficient. This screen is of the software program mCalc.

Let's continue with this example, this time examining what happens when the bone-conduction threshold is not 0 dB, but turns out to be 30 dB HL. (Figure 9-11.) Continuing with the case above, the audiologist had assumed a 0 dB right bone-conduction threshold, and used 45 dB EM based on the "MMax" approach to formula masking. The right ear bone-conduction threshold was measured at 30 dB HL. The minimum level = 30 + 20 dB NTE ABG + 10 dB safety pad = 60 dB EM. The 45 dB calculated MMax is causing undermasking. As shown in Figure 9-11, with the knowledge that the test ear bone-conduction threshold is actually 30, the MMax is 75 dB EM.

Chapter 9. Formula Masking – Bone Conduction

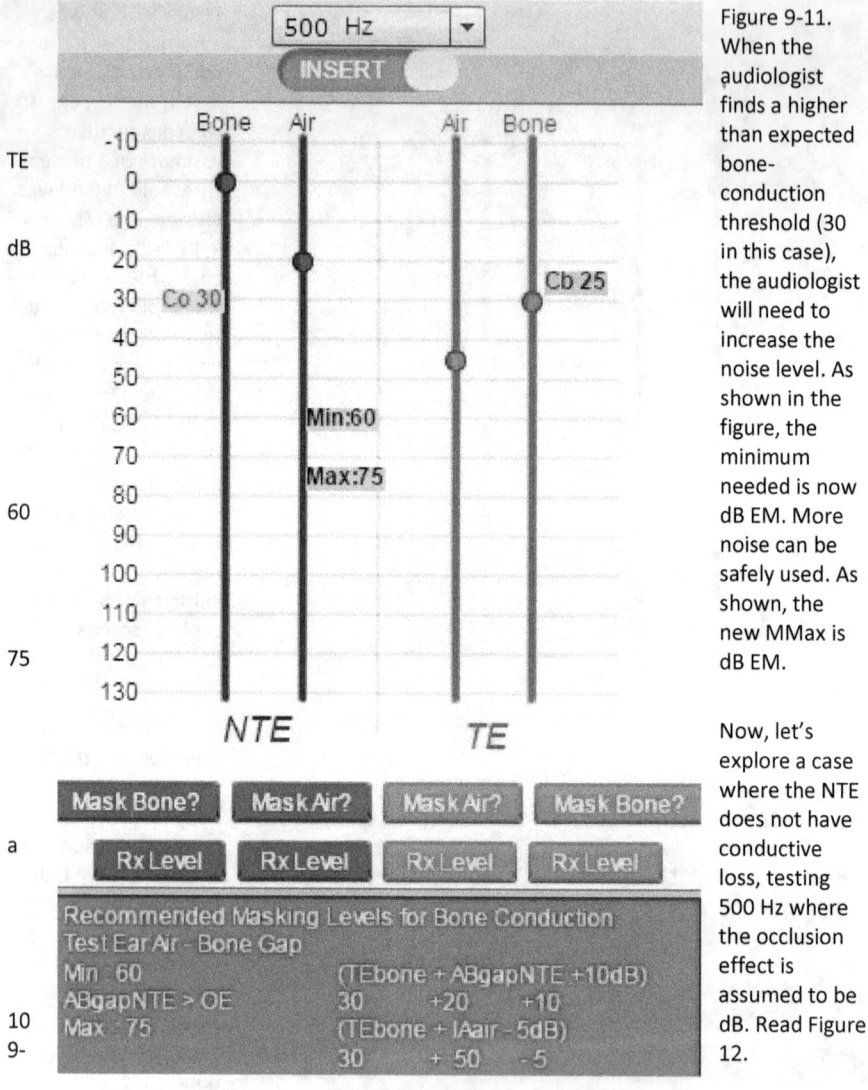

Figure 9-11. When the audiologist finds a higher than expected bone-conduction threshold (30 in this case), the audiologist will need to increase the noise level. As shown in the figure, the minimum needed is now dB EM. More noise can be safely used. As shown, the new MMax is dB EM.

Now, let's explore a case where the NTE does not have conductive loss, testing 500 Hz where the occlusion effect is assumed to be dB. Read Figure 9-12.

Chapter 9. Formula Masking – Bone Conduction

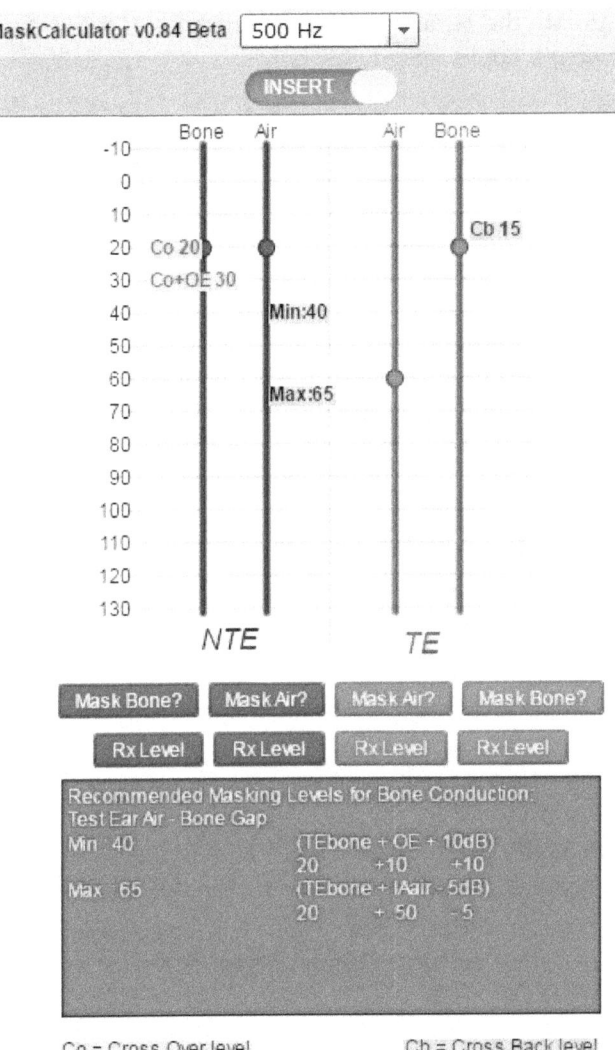

Figure 9-12. The conservative estimation is that the right ear's bone-conduction threshold is 20 dB HL – the same as the better ear's threshold (which was measured first, without contralateral masking). The MMax approach ensures you are not overmasking, as long as threshold is not better than you estimated. After obtaining threshold (e.g. it is as predicted at 20 dB HL), then calculate the minimum masking level, using the occlusion effect value in this example, because there is no NTE air-bone gap. MMin is < MMax, so masking is sufficient and overmasking is not a concern.

Step-by-Step Approach to Using the "MMax" Formula Masking Approach

You may well understand the process, but in case you could use the redundancy, here's a review of the steps in using the MMax process.

Step one. Estimate the bone-conduction threshold of the test ear as the lowest it could reasonably be.

Use the most conservative (lowest) bone-conduction threshold estimate as your basis for finding the maximum safe masking level. If you suspect conductive loss, and if you have an unmasked bone-conduction threshold, use that level. If you have not obtained the unmasked threshold but believe the loss is conductive, then use 0 dB HL (or even -10 dB HL).

If you are fairly sure that there is some cochlear loss, then think about the LEAST amount of loss that may be present, and use that as your estimate. For example, if I am retesting a patient and have the prior audiogram, with no reason to think that hearing has improved (though it may have worsened), I would choose a level a bit lower than what was found at the last evaluation. I would not use exactly the level found last time, as thresholds vary +/- 5 dB from test to retest. A level 10 dB below that found last time would be a good starting point. If I believe the loss is sensorineural, I could use the air-conduction threshold or preferably 10-20 dB below that level. (Because the MMax process uses a 50 dB interaural attenuation value, and your patient's interaural attenuation value is likely more, it's not imperative that you use the 10 dB below value but it's likely to save you time. You won't have to consider overmasking if the BC threshold is slightly lower than the AC threshold.)

If air-conduction testing has indicated a severe loss, and you anticipate that you will be recording a "no response" at the audiometer output limits, technically MMax is still based upon the cochlear sensitivity, and will yield a very high masking intensity. Subsituting the output limits of the bone-conduction transducer yields a more reasonable MMax. (Regardless of what the calculated value is, do not use a masking level that would create loudness discomfort.)

If you are wrong, and the threshold is better than that, you'll need to recalculate. (It's not the end of the world!)

Step two. Add 45 dB. Use that contralateral masking noise level to establish the actual bone-conduction threshold.

Using your usual Hughson-Westlake threshold seeking approach, find the masked bone-conduction threshold. If you previously established the unmasked threshold, you can check for hearing at that level with masking, and if the tone is still heard, then you don't need to re-establish threshold. However, the threshold will probably be at least 5 dB higher, due to the central masking effect.

Step three. Double check that the threshold was no lower than what you estimated. (Check for possible overmasking.)

When using the MMax approach, if the threshold is lower than expected, you may have overmasking.

Overmasking may be occurring

If BC threshold + 45 < MMax

For example, if you guessed a 20 dB HL bone-conduction threshold, which gives you the Mmax calculation of 65 dB EM, and the real threshold is 10 dB HL, you may have overmasked. 10 dB BC threshold + 45 = 55 which is lower than your MMax level of 65 dB EM. (65 dB EM can cross back to the test ear and can potentially prevent hearing of tones at or lower than 15 dB HL.) If this occurs, then use the new threshold in calculating the new, lower MMax level to use. Estimate that threshold is at least 10 dB better than what you are measuring so that, in case it was overmasking.

Another way to think about potential overmasking:

If MMax - 50 ≥ TE BC

Overmasking may be occurring

Why 45 above and 50 here? It's about less/greater than and equal to! you are OK if the noise is 45 dB above the NTE threshold; you are not OK if it is 50 dB above, or even higher intensity. Adding and subtracting even numbers is easier, so this is my preferred way of checking for overmasking.

Step four. Check that the masking level was adequate. (Check for undermasking)

You should always do this check, but it's particularly important if the BC threshold is coming in higher than you guessed. After measuring the bone-conduction threshold using the MMax approach, calculate the minimum masking level with the usual formula, using the threshold you just established.

Minimum Masking Level =

BC threshold + (Larger of OE or NTE ABG) + 10 dB.

Ensure that MMax was greater than or equal to the minimum level. If this is not the case, then you are undermasking. If you find that you don't have enough masking noise, you need to use more noise to mask the crossover, or you may need to plateau mask. Sometimes you can combine a bit of plateau masking to your formula masking. If the noise level at the cochlea (Noise-NTE ABG/OE) is only slightly higher than the TE BC threshold, then you should increase the noise slightly and check that the tone is still audible. (If not, then raising the noise either overmasked or it was previously undermasked. Remember, "If in doubt, plateau it out.")

If the reason that you need more masking is that the bone-conduction threshold turned out to be higher than you assumed, then recalculating the MMax and finding threshold again should let you measure threshold correctly. However, if the bone-conduction threshold is similar to what you guessed, and you are observing air-bone gaps, then you can't formula mask – you may (or may not) have a masking dilemma. Abandon the formula masking approach: plateau mask this frequency.

mQuest Level 19

The next level steps you through the MMax procedures. In level 19 the non-test ear does not have air-bone gaps: Use the occlusion effect in calculating MMax.

Chapter 9. Formula Masking – Bone Conduction

Which Approach: Min or Max?

Max is Best with TE Conductive Loss

Which approach is best to use, Min or Max? It depends on your patient and your suspicion of site of lesion. If the patient complains of otalgia, hearing loss co-occurring with a cold, and/or has abnormal immittance findings, then you suspect conductive loss (or conductive overlay) and using the "Max" approach is more likely to work best for you.

Min is Nice for TE SNHL – Less Intense Noise Used

If in the history taking your patient tells you "I can hear fine in quiet, but I'm having difficulty in noisy environments, and increasingly I have to use the phone on this ear" then you are suspecting asymmetrical, probably sensorineural, loss. The "Min" approach will likely be efficient and it will use lower levels of masking noise, which would be more comfortable for your patient. You can use MMax, but be sure not to cause loudness discomfort.

Guess a Low BC TE Threshold if Using the MMax and Guess High When Using MMin

With the minimum masking approach, best for sensorineural losses, you make a guess of threshold, and you should guess that the bone-conduction threshold is as bad as it can get: i.e., equal to the air-conduction level or the audiometer maximum output level, whichever is lower. If the test ear threshold turns out to be worse than you expected, then the minimum isn't enough. That's why you use the "worst case scenario" (guess a high bone-conduction threshold) with the Min approach. If your guess turns out to be wrong, and the loss has a conductive element, and thus the bone-conduction threshold is significantly better than your estimate, then it is imperative that you check to see if you have overmasked. That gets us back to why you may favor MMin for the sensorineural losses, but MMax when the test ear has conductive loss.

With the MMax (maximum safe level to use) approach, best for conductive and mixed loss, you limit the noise intensity to prevent overmasking. Guess the lowest reasonably possible bone-conduction threshold. If your guess is wrong (the bone-conduction is better than even what you guessed), you'll have to reduce the noise level. Guessing low in the first place reduces that chance. But, guessing too low increases the likelihood that your check that you have enough masking noise shows that you don't, and you have to increase the noise level. If "max" was calculated based on too low a threshold, the true bone-conduction threshold is higher, then you may have crossover that isn't completely masked.

You can switch back and forth between the approaches if you need to recalculate.

Plateau Mask if MMin > MMax with the Same Estimated Threshold

If in doing your MMin / MMax double checks you find that the minimum either is the same as the maximum, or worse, is higher than MMax, then it's time to plateau mask if that is possible. For this rule to work, both MMin and MMax need to be based on the same threshold. (Normally you would guess low for MMin and high for MMax, this rule doesn't work if you do that.)

For example, the NTE has a 35 dB air-bone gap and the TE has a 20 dB air-bone gap and a 15 dB HL bone-conduction threshold in preliminary testing.

- MMin = 15 + 35 NTE ABG + 10 pad = 60
- MMax = 15 + 45 = 60

It would be safest to plateau, but technically you can formula mask. You are using the maximum before risking overmasking, if the interaural attenuation is 50 dB.

What if you can't plateau? (This will come up in the next chapter – with word recognition testing, plateau is not an option.) I would advocate using the minimum level. Since the interaural attenuation is likely higher than 50, you probably won't overmask. Annotating the results (making a note in the report) would be appropriate.

Hmmm, what would I write? "It should be noted that formula masking was used (due to… e.g. the limited attention span of the child), which is sub-optimal. Thresholds may be elevated by overmasking if the patient's interaural attenuation is at the minimum amount clinically observed."

Test Bone-Conduction at the Lowest Frequency First. Use One Frequency's Threshold to Guess the Next Threshold

Students are taught to test air-conduction at 1000 Hz first, in the better ear. That's perfectly sensible advice. Obviously test the better ear, if there is one, first so that when you switch to the poorer hearing ear, you will know if you need to mask. Testing 1000 Hz first is good because it approximates what patients would expect to hear when you tell them to press the button when the "tone" is heard: starting at 250 Hz (which may sound like a fog horn) or 8000 Hz (a squeak, which may be inaudible with sloping sensorineural hearing loss) would potentially confuse the patient. However, once you've tested the patient across the range of frequencies, that confusion is removed. The patient knows what the test tones will be. So here's a suggestion. When you test bone-conduction, START AT THE LOWEST FREQUENCY FIRST.

If the loss is sensorineural at the lowest frequency, it is likely to be sensorineural at the other frequencies as well. The "minimum masking level" approach is likely to be efficient and exposes the patient to the lowest possible noise levels. Conversely, if you find conductive or mixed loss, you may want to use the "max" approach. In this case, the low-frequency bone-conduction threshold will also help you make an estimate of the hearing at the higher frequencies. (Since hearing loss is often sloping, bone-conduction thresholds are usually the same or worse at the higher frequencies.)

One Last mQuest Game Level

You are ready for the final Quest. Tackle level 20. Cases have air-bone gaps in the test ear, the non-test ear, or both. Are you ready? [What is your professor's best time on this level? As of this writing, mine is 359 seconds (without by-passing the step of guessing the threshold)].

Using the Masking Calculator – mCalc

Another software program, called mCalc, is available: http://www.audstudent.com/mcalc. mCalc has a couple of potential uses. You could use it in the clinic as you are learning formula masking to help coach you. You can also use it now, if there are some ideas that you are not quite clear on.

Chapter 9. Formula Masking – Bone Conduction

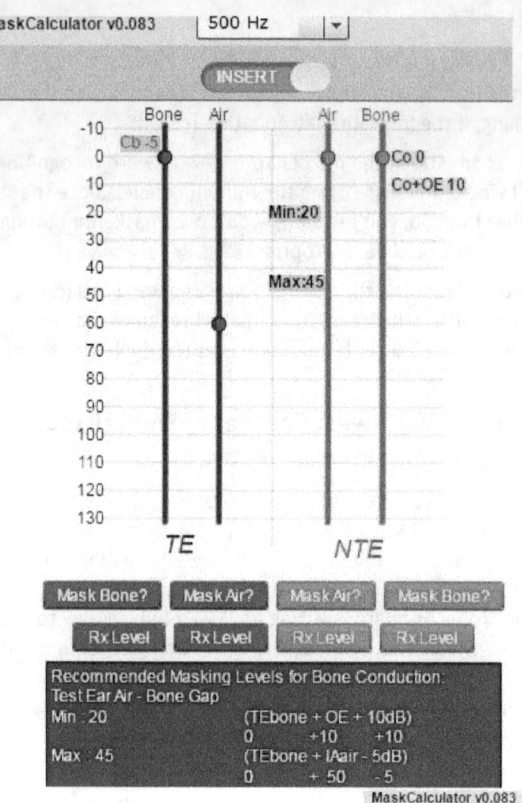

Input the expected thresholds by adjusting the sliders. The calculator's "Rx Level" will show the MMin and MMax, using the formulas described in this chapter. See Figure 9-13 and 9-14 below.

Figure 9-13. Clicking "Rx Level" below the test ear (TE) "Mask Bone?" box shows the MMin and MMax values graphically, with the formulas shown below.

Figure 9-14. Note that the NTE has an air-bone gap, and the formula (see bottom blue box) substitutes that ABGap for the OE value.

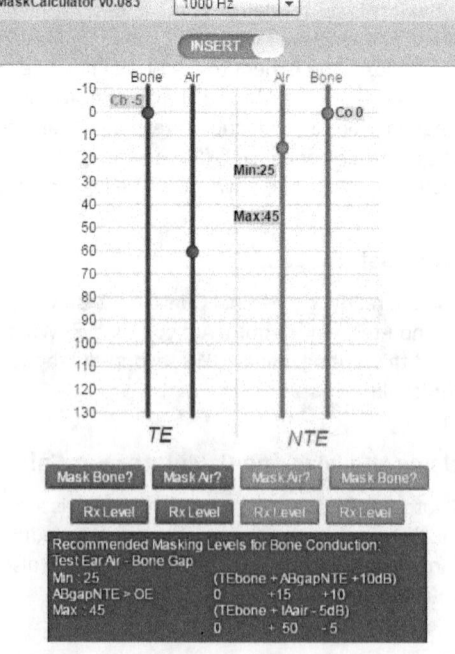

Chapter 9. Formula Masking – Bone Conduction

KEY CONCEPTS

Steps for Finding Bone-Conduction Minimum Masking Level (MMin)

1. Estimate the bone-conduction threshold of the test ear. This is the starting point of your bone-conduction masking formula. Be pessimistic in your guess – guess high.

2. Add a 10 dB "safety pad".

3. Add the larger of the occlusion effect size or the NTE conductive hearing loss size.

4. Apply this level noise to the non-test ear and establish/confirm hearing threshold.

5. Check whether the measured threshold you obtained is at or lower than the value you used as your estimate when making the formula masking calculation. If it is, you are not undermasking. Next, check for overmasking.

6. Determine if overmasking may have made your results invalid. Note the noise level that you used. Subtract 50 dB – the minimum interaural attenuation value for insert earphones. If the bone-conduction threshold you just measured is at that level or lower (less impairment), then your results may have been influenced by overmasking. If so, recalculate the noise level and re-establish threshold.

7. If the bone-conduction threshold is higher than anticipated, check to ensure that you are not undermasking. Recalculate MMin and use this masking level -- re-establish threshold

8. If you have neither over- nor undermasked, then mark your threshold and move on to the next test frequency.

Chapter 9. Formula Masking – Bone Conduction

Steps for Finding Bone-Conduction Maximum Masking Level (MMax)

1. Calculate MMax: lowest anticipated bone conduction threshold + 45 dB.

2. Check that you are not undermasking. Undermasking is a problem when the measured BC threshold is higher than estimated.

> ▪ Calculate MMin once you know the bone-conduction threshold
>
> Minimum Masking level = BC threshold + (Larger of OE or NTE ABG) + 10 dB.
>
> If MMax is lower than MMin, then you do not have sufficient masking. Switch to the Minimum Masking Formula and use the threshold you just measured, which was higher than what you had estimated as the bone-conduction threshold when you calculated the Maximum Masking Level.

3. Check that the measured threshold is not lower than you initially guessed. If it was, you may be overmasking. Recalculate MMax and check threshold again with that lower noise level.

4. If you are not overmasking, not undermasking, then you are done. Mark threshold – next frequency, please!

Chapter 10

Formula Masking for Speech Stimuli

Formulae Quick Reference

Spondee Threshold Minimum Masking Level:
Predicted SPONDEE THRESHOLD + 10 dB in case the SPONDEE THRESHOLD is a bit higher than the PTA predicts – IA (60 dB for inserts, 50 for TDH) + largest significant NTE ABG + 10 dB pad
Insert Earphones ⇒ TE estimated SPONDEE THRESHOLD – 40 dB + Largest significant NTE ABG (500 Hz to 8k Hz)
Supra-aural Phones ⇒ TE estimated SPONDEE THRESHOLD – 30 dB + Largest significant NTE ABG (500 Hz to 8k Hz)

Word Recognition Testing Minimum Masking Level:
Presentation level – IA + 10 dB pad + Largest significant NTE ABG (500 Hz to 8k Hz)
Insert Earphones ⇒ TE signal level – 50 dB + NTE ABG dB + Largest Significant NTE ABG (500 Hz to 8k Hz)
For Supra-aural Phones ⇒ TE signal level – 40 dB + Largest Significant NTE ABG ABG (500 Hz to 8k Hz)

Maximum Masking Level
For both spondee threshold and word recognition testing: Best TE BC threshold in the 500-8k Hz range + IA – 5
For insert earphone ⇒ Best TE 500 to 8k Hz + 55 dB
For Supra-aural Phones ⇒ BC TE 500 to 8k Hz + 45 dB
For safety, assume the best bone is 10 dB lower than AC thresholds for sensorineural loss and 0 dB for conductive losses.

Down 20 Rule:
Estimated spondee threshold or word recognition test level – 20 dB.
Simple, easy to calculate, and works well for asymmetrical sensorineural loss. If the test ear has conductive loss, this rule could lead to some overmasking, but it is usually not consequential – it won't typically interfere with speech understanding. Non-test ear conductive loss may cause this rule to undermask.

Some crossback is not the end of the world. Crossback to the TE cochlea is not going to interfere with hearing speech that is 10 dB or more greater than the crossback level. Calculate the sensation level of the stimulus at the test ear (and do this across the frequency ranges). Calculate the sensation level of the crossback at the test ear (again, across frequencies). If the stimulus is 10 dB or more greater than the crossback, then your results are not significantly affected by the crossback.

Chapter 10. Speech Masking

Speech Testing Introduction

Congratulations on making it this far into formula masking. The chapter on "why formula mask" discussed that when conducting speech testing, especially word recognition testing, you need to formula mask. You can't plateau. So everything you have learned so far will now be applied where you need it most.

Speech masking requires one more cognitive stretch. You'll have to think about hearing sensitivity all the frequencies, since speech and speech noise are wide-band stimuli.

The formula masking concepts remain the same. You need to ensure that you have enough noise at the NTE cochlea to mask any crossover. Now, we'll add in that means thinking about cross over at each frequency. You'll need to increase that noise level if the NTE has significant air-bone gaps. You need to ensure that the masking noise isn't going to cross back at a level that will interfere with speech understanding. Here's where you get a little leeway. If there is just a little crossback, but the speech signal is well above that crossback level, then the crossback won't significantly affect the speech test results. You are still looking at the test ear bone-conduction thresholds, and basing your MMax calculations on them. Of course, usually you do speech testing via air-conduction before you test bone-conduction hearing, so you have to make an educated guess about the bone-conduction thresholds.

There is a simple formula masking rule that is going to work most of the time. You examine your presentation level, and simply put in contralateral noise that is 20 dB less intense. That's called the "Down 20" rule. The good news is that works for asymmetrical sensorineural losses, which constitutes the bulk of the cases seen in a general audiology practice. The bad news is that it won't work with significant conductive loss, so you need to read and understand the entire chapter.

So, without further delay, let's delve right in.

Speech Interaural Attenuation Value: 60 dB for insert earphones, 50 dB for TDH

Given how often masking for speech is conducted, we have surprisingly little data on the appropriate interaural attenuation (IA) value when using insert earphones. A literature search reveals one study – by Sklare and Denenberg (1987). They tested seven (yes, count them, seven!) patients with unilateral profound hearing loss and found that the average insert earphone interaural attenuation value was 75 dB, the minimum was 70. With only seven subjects, the true minimum is likely below 70 dB. They reported that the standard deviation was 7 dB; so the 2 standard deviation limit that should encompass 98% of the population predicts that the minimum IA is 61 dB, which we'll round to 60 dB.

There are more data available re: TDH-style earphones. The minimum IA value is 48 dB in most literature. We can "afford" to round that up to 50 dB so long as we are using a 10 dB "pad" – a little extra in case of calibration errors or in case we are testing those with extremely low interaural attenuation. Remember this slight "cheat" in considering when to mask – err on the side of caution.

Chapter 10. Speech Masking

The Acoustics of Speech, the Acoustics of Interaural Attenuation

How loud is speech at each 1/3 octave band? Where is the bulk of the speech energy? Table 10-1 shows data from Cox and Moore (1988) – there is more energy in the average speaker's voice in the low frequencies (long term average, of speaker with overall level of 70 dB SPL). Conveniently and coincidentally, the insert earphone interaural attenuation values are greater in the low frequencies. Table 10-1 shows the lowest minimum IA values for the published studies reviewed. This is good news. Where there is more speech energy, there is more interaural attenuation, so we can treat the crossover as being equal intensity level across the frequencies.

Table 10-1. Although speech has greater low-frequency energy, insert earphones have greater low-frequency interaural attenuation. The net result is that air-conduction speech will be at a relatively even level across the frequency range when it reaches the non-test ear cochlea.

Frequency (Hz)	250	500	1k	2k	4k	8k
Spectrum Level of Speech Energy (dB SPL)	60	62	55	49	46	45
Interaural Attenuation Minimum (dB)	63	62	56	50	50	60

Check Need for Masking – Is the Crossover Above NTE Bone-Conduction Thresholds in the 500 to 8k Hz Range?

In determining the need for masking for spondee threshold or word recognition testing, consider if any of the speech energy could be heard, by bone-conduction, in the non-test ear. Examine the range from 500 Hz to 8000 Hz. Why not 250 Hz?

When formula masking spondee thresholds, we need to consider which frequencies contribute to the hearing of the words. Generally, hearing only 250 Hz energy would not be enough to permit one to differentiate which spondee was presented. But, hearing at essentially any other frequency could permit speech understanding. (Hearing at 250 Hz will contribute to the spondee understanding, however. It will aid in vowel recognition.) Word understanding of monosyllabic words also won't occur just if hearing 250 Hz.

If obtaining a speech detection threshold, then even 250 Hz hearing should be considered: Detection requires only audibility.

The patient with an audiogram shown in Figure 10-1 may have a right ear 120 dB HL spondee threshold (if the audiometer output goes that high), or may have no recognition at all – that's pretty likely given the cochlear distortions that a hearing loss of that magnitude would create.

Chapter 10. Speech Masking

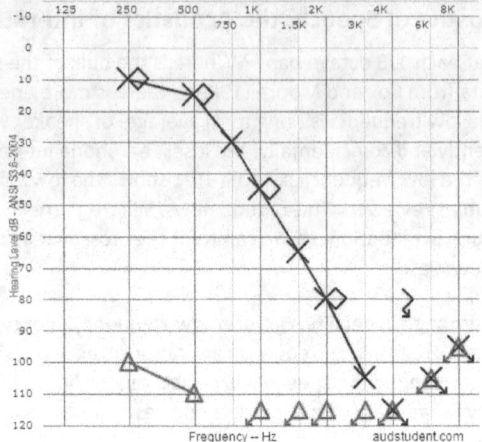

Figure 10-1. You would not expect the patient to recognize spondee words in the right ear when properly masked, but you would attempt testing so that your results are complete. Assume that the audiometer output can test as high as 120 dB HL.

We would calculate the need for masking based upon the assumption that the interaural attenuation is 60 dB. If 120 dB HL speech can be presented, then we need to consider -- would the non-test ear hear the crossover (by bone conduction)? Figure 10-2 illustrates.

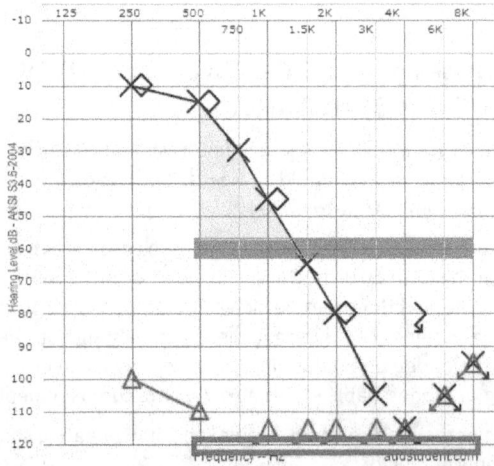

Figure 10-2. In the worst-case scenario, the interaural attenuation would be as little as 60 dB for speech, so words presented at 120 dB HL could be audible by bone-conduction at the areas of the cochlea encoding ~1350 Hz and lower frequencies. Examine the best bone-conduction threshold – if the cross hearing is possible at any frequency, 500-8k Hz, then masking is warranted. Masking is needed in this example. The crossover can be detected in the NTE at the cochlea, using the 500 Hz and 1k Hz places.

Chapter 10. Speech Masking

Word Recognition Supra-Threshold Testing Frequently Requires Masking

Pure-tone masking has trained the eye to recognize that large interaural differences signal the need for masking. You'll need to learn new strategies in order to not miss the need for speech masking. You will need to think about the presentation level – and compare that to the non-test ear's best bone-conduction thresholds. Because you are testing at a level that is well above threshold, and well above the non-test ear bone-conduction thresholds, you will frequently need to mask.

Word Recognition Cross-Hearing – Detection Alone May Not Permit Open-Set Word Recognition. Consider the Sensation Level

It's easier (requires less hearing) to repeat spondee words from a list of a handful of choices than it is to correctly recognize what word was presented during word recognition testing. So for word recognition testing, a little bit of crossover might not truly improve the word recognition score. However, audiologists tend to be cautious and if there is any possibility of the non-test ear participating then contralateral masking is used. This means sometimes we will mask when it wasn't essential. Figure 10-3 offers an example where the minimal cross hearing during word recognition testing does not do much to aid in figuring out which word was heard. Very little speech energy would be heard in the left ear. If this patient scored even modestly well (e.g. perhaps 40% or better), without contralateral masking having been used, then I would doubt that the non-test ear hearing (alone) could explain that score. Consider the degree to which the speech could be suprathreshold in the non-test ear. If it is marginal, as in Figure 10-3, then it is not an aid to word recognition. However, it doesn't hurt to mask to eliminate any possibility that the non-test ear is contributing to the word recognition.

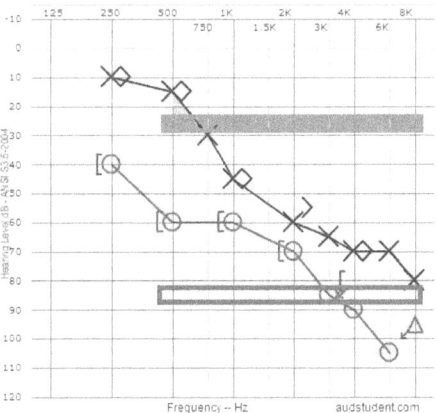

Figure 10-3. There is no need to mask for right ear spondee testing. The expected spondee threshold is about 60 dB HL. Crossover would be at 0 dB HL and inaudible. However, if testing word recognition at 85 dB HL in the right ear, the crossover (25 dB HL) is audible. Masking should be conducted, but a very low word recognition score would be expected if only the cross-hearing is contributing to word understanding. Only the speech energy below ~600 Hz is audible in the non-test (left) ear cochlea.

High-Intensity Speech Testing (e.g. Rollover Testing) Requires Masking (Sometimes Even Without Significant Asymmetry)

Audiologists may test word recognition at high intensity levels in order to determine if word recognition performance is poor or has decreased when intensity was increased – a sign of potential retrocochlear involvement. Since high test stimulus levels are used, crossover is high; participation of the contralateral ear would invalidate test results. Figure 10-4 illustrates.

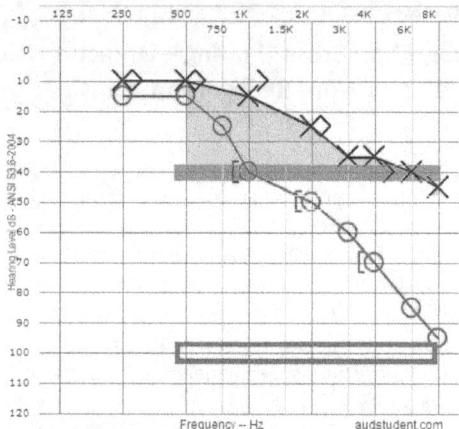

Figure 10-4. Crossover of the right ear 100 dB HL speech signal to the non-test (left) ear could significantly improve the word recognition score. Even though the asymmetry is not large, masking when testing word recognition at high intensities is necessary.

Even with symmetrical hearing, high intensity speech testing requires masking. Even if the right ear in the audiogram in Figure 10-4 had the same hearing as the left ear, if word recognition were assessed at 100 dB HL, there will be the same crossover to the non-test ear

Spondee Threshold Masking

Recognizing the Need for Masking Summarized

Estimate spondee threshold, add 10 dB. Subtract 60 dB (IA for insert earphones). If this is above the possible bone-conduction thresholds 500 – 8k Hz, then masking is needed.

- To be efficient with spondee threshold formula masking, you want to make sure that you are masking when needed "from the start." If you obtain the unmasked spondee threshold, then recognize the need for masking, you have to do extra testing. To avoid this possibility, consider the highest spondee threshold you would expect. The two-frequency average plus about 10 dB would be a good estimate. You want to go 10 dB "above" your estimate so that, if the spondee threshold is a bit higher than your estimate, you don't have to go back and mask.

- Subtract 60 dB, the interaural attenuation value (for insert earphones, 50 for TDH).

Chapter 10. Speech Masking

- Compare this level to the non-test ear bone-conduction thresholds at 500 to 8k Hz (include 250 Hz if obtaining a speech detection threshold). If the probable bone-conduction thresholds are lower – you need to mask.
- If immittance is normal, use the NTE air-conduction thresholds as your guide for whether masking is needed. To be safest, consider the "what if" – what if the bone-conduction threshold is 10 dB lower? Use that as your estimate, again, so that you don't obtain the unmasked threshold, then after obtaining bone-conduction thresholds, realize that you did have to mask. If immittance is abnormal and/or symptoms suggest conductive involvement, then most likely you would assume 0 dB HL bone-conduction thresholds, or perhaps even lower if the patient is young.

Formula for Min Mask: Expected Spondee Threshold – 40 dB (for inserts) + Largest Significant NTE Air-Bone Gap

As with formula masking for pure tones, guessing the threshold will help you be efficient during testing. The pure-tone average should help you predict the spondee threshold you will eventually obtain. To reiterate, you won't want to use exactly the predicted threshold in your minimum masking formula. If threshold comes in even a little higher, that would mean you have undermasked, and would need to increase the masking level. It is better to build the "what if the spondee threshold is a bit higher than estimated" into the formula.

Masking noise presented to the non-test ear is attenuated by any conductive loss in that non-test ear, so if you have any reason to believe there is conductive loss, estimate it (and use the worst case scenario – that it is as large as it could realistically be.) Add that into the minimum masking formula. As for pure-tone testing, if the air-bone gap is the 5 dB or so air-bone gap that is due to test-retest variability, those don't need to be accounted for. When immittance is abnormal, then you should be very concerned, and the safest course is to assume bone-conduction thresholds are normal and calculate the air-bone gap. (As with pure-tone masking, you might want to switch to a MMax approach.)

Minimum Masking Level = Expected SPONDEE THRESHOLD + 10 in case it's a bit higher + 10 for pad – 60 for IA + the largest significant NTE air-bone gap at any frequency 500-8k Hz.

This formula simplifies to: **Expected Spondee Threshold – 40 dB (for inserts) + Largest Significant NTE Air-Bone Gap**

TDH: Since the IA value is 10 dB lower, it would be SPONDEE THRESHOLD – 30 + Largest ABG (500 to 8 kHz)

Formula for Max Mask (both Spondee Threshold and Word Recognition): Best TE BC threshold from 500 to 8k Hz + 55 dB

How much masking is absolutely safe? If none of the crossback is audible, that is ideal. Assume a 60 dB IA at each frequency.

We can safely present up to 55 dB above the best bone-conduction threshold. If we go all the way up to 60 we risk some crossback interference.

So, the formula is **MMax = Best TE bone-conduction threshold (500 to 8 kHz) + 55 dB**

This formula holds the same for both spondee threshold and for word recognition testing, but as an upcoming section will discuss, a little bit of cross back may not hurt. As long as the speech signal is well above the crossback, the speech is still audible.

Chapter 10. Speech Masking

When thinking about the potential crossback and the number to use as "Best TE bone threshold", think about cochlear sensitivity rather than the maximum output of the audiometer. For example, in Figure 10-5 below, the cochlear sensitivity at 500 Hz is probably 80 dB HL, which is higher than the audiometer bone-conduction circuit can produce. (Overmasking is dictated by the noise interfering with the test ear's hearing, so that is what we need to consider. You won't have overmasking unless the crossback is 80 dB or higher.) It would be a good idea to consider the possibility of a slight conductive loss, however. If you wish to be "extra safe" you could use 10 dB below the guessed best bone-conduction threshold.

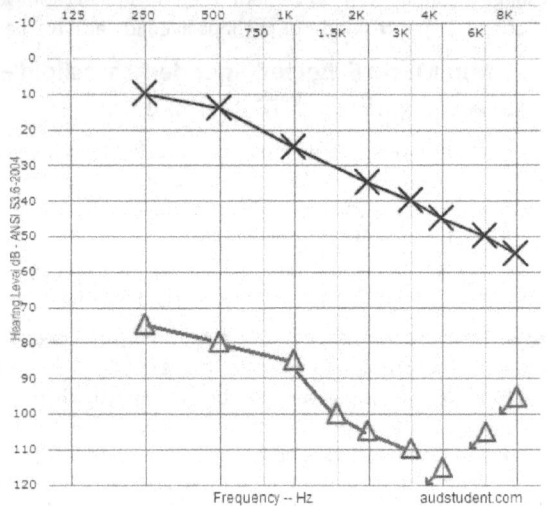

Figure 10-5. Assume that the loss is sensorineural in each ear. The estimated spondee threshold is about 85 dB HL. Masking is needed: Crossover could be 25 dB HL and audible at 500 and 1000 Hz.

Review – Example

Let's calculate MMIn and MMax for the case shown in Figure 10-5.

MMin = Expected Spondee Threshold (85 dB HL) + 10 (ST could be 95 dB HL) – IA (60 dB) + 10 dB pad.

The short form is MMin = 85 – 40 = 45 dB EM.

MMax = Best test ear BC threshold that could be found in the 500-8k range (80 dB HL), but for safety, calculate MMax based on a threshold that is 10 dB lower than what I really think the cochlear sensitivity will be. MMax = 70 dB HL + 55 = 125 dB EM.

T

To reiterate, the maximum formula has us look at the 80 dB 500 Hz threshold, yielding a maximum of 135 dB EM. But let's use a true worst case scenario. Maybe there is a slight conductive overlay – cochlear sensitivity might be as good as 70 dB HL. 70 plus 55 dB: 125 dB EM – a level at or above the audiometer's output and a level that would be intolerably loud and grossly inappropriate! (Remember, this is going into the left ear which has normal low-frequency hearing and high-frequency recruitment.)

The "Down 20" Formula

There is a simple formula that works well when the loss in each ear is sensorineural. It simply advocates that you estimated the spondee threshold, and use contralateral noise that is 20 dB lower than this level. That will give you a value between minimum and maximum when you have sensorineural hearing loss. You don't have to guess the spondee threshold as being higher, but do consider that if the need for masking is borderline, it is better to mask when it's possibly needed. This will prevent you from having to come back and mask should the spondee threshold come in a bit higher than the pure-tone average.

As will be further discussed below, if there is conductive loss in the non-test ear (which lowers the effectiveness of the contralateral masking), this formula may lead you to undermask. When there is conductive loss in the test ear, your stimulation will be loud, and your contralateral masking also needs to be more intense. More intense masking noise means a greater likelihood of crossback. There is a chance of crossback that can go unrecognized with the simple "Down 20" formula. Generally though, to have overmasking the conductive loss needs to be greater that the loss severity that one typically sees.

There is nothing magical about the 20 dB number. Preceptors may prefer a "Down 25" or "Down 30" formula.

In Figure 10-5, MMin = 45 dB EM; MMax = 125 dB EM. "Down 20" for the expected 85 dB HL spondee threshold indicates use of 65 dB EM. Isn't that a lot easier! But remember – the Down 20 Formula works well for bilateral sensorineural loss, but not as well for conductive loss, as the sections below will describe further.

Spondee Threshold Testing Examples
Asymmetrical Sensorineural Loss Example Reviewed Again

Let's examine another case of asymmetrical sensorineural loss. See Figure 10-6 and its legend.

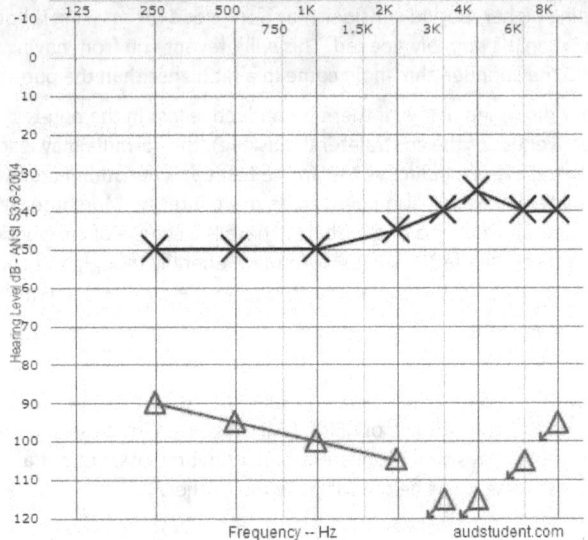

Figure 10-6. Assume that this loss is sensorineural bilaterally. **MMin** for spondee threshold testing = 100 dB HL – 40 = **60 dB EM. MMax** = 85 dB HL (the 500 Hz bone-conduction threshold of 95 that you would measure if your audiometer let you test at that high an intensity, minus 10 dB in case cochlear sensitivity is slightly better than anticipated) + 55 = the ludicrously loud **140** dB EM. The **Down 20 rule** would recommend use of **80 dB EM.**

NTE Conductive Loss Spondee Threshold Masking Example

Non-test ear conductive loss reduces the effectiveness of masking noise, raising the minimum masking level. This can cause the "Down 20" formula to undermask. Figure 10-7 illustrates.

Chapter 10. Speech Masking

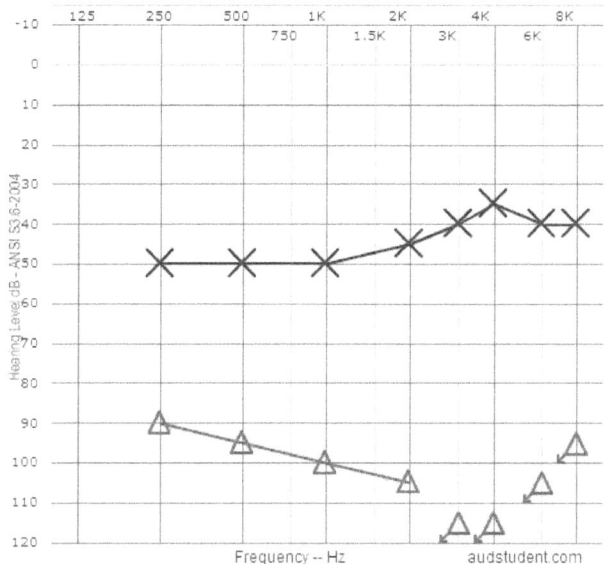

Figure 10-7 Assume that immittance is consistent with left ear conductive loss, and prior audiometric testing indicated that the right ear loss is sensorineural. The NTE largest air-bone gap (at 500 to 8k Hz) is assumed to be 50 dB. (If you want to make it 60 dB, that's not wrong.)

The **minimum masking formula** = Expected spondee threshold (~100) – 40 + 50 ABG = **110 dB EM**. While that is loud, remember that not all of the sound is audible – it is attenuated by the non-test ear conductive loss

The **maximum masking level** is again the stratospheric 85 dB (best reasonably expected cochlear hearing sensitivity anticipated in the right ear, estimated as 10 dB better than the 500 Hz AC threshold) + 55 = **140 dB EM.**

The **Down 20** level – expected 100 dB spondee threshold minus 20 dB – is **80 dB EM**. This illustrates that **the Down 20 formula can lead to undermasking with NTE conductive loss.** The 80 dB EM is lower than the 110 required to minimally mask the left ear

Test Ear Conductive Loss Spondee Threshold Examples

When the test ear loss is conductive, overmasking becomes a concern, and the "Down 20" formula may lead you to overmask. Refer to Figure 10-8.

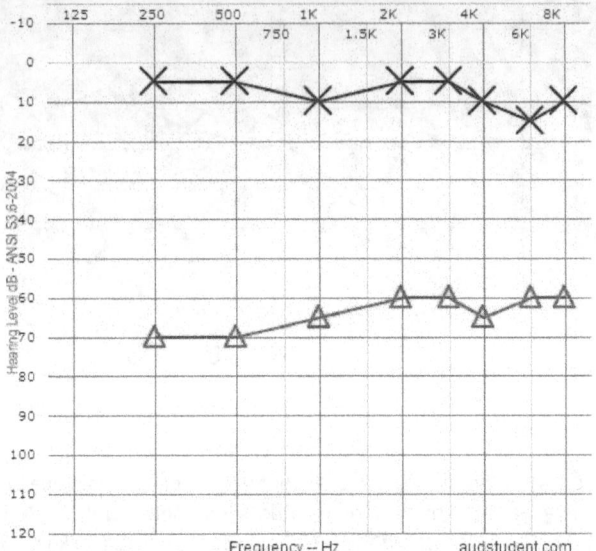

Figure 10-8. Assume that the patient's symptoms and immittance results are consistent with the finding of conductive loss in the right ear.

The **minimum masking level** is ~65 dB expected SPONDEE THRESHOLD – 40 = **25 dB EM**.

The **maximum masking level** could be assumed to be 5 dB (best bone-conduction threshold) or 0 dB (if you want to be even more conservative) + 55: either **60 or 55 dB EM**. Any level between 25 and 55/60 dB EM would adequately mask.

The **Down 20** rule calls for 45 dB EM. This falls within the range of minimum and maximum. A more extreme test ear conductive loss is shown in Figure 10-9.

Chapter 10. Speech Masking

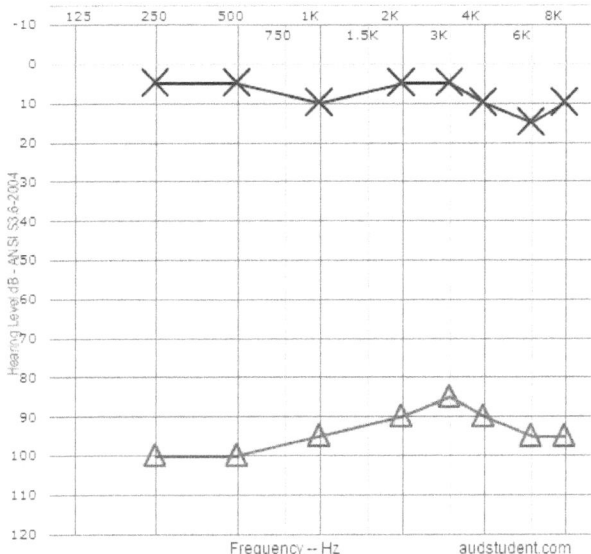

Figure 10-9. To have a right ear conductive loss this severe would be rare – perhaps a congenital absence of a middle ear cavity and/or atresia (that still magically allows you to use insert earphones).

The **minimum** masking level is the estimated spondee threshold (~95 dB HL) – 40 = 55.

Assuming that bone-conduction threshold is 5 dB, perhaps 0 dB HL, giving a **maximum masking level of 55-60 dB EM**. Note the very narrow range between minimum and maximum with this truly maximal conductive loss in the test ear.

The **Down 20** formula would call for **75 dB EM, which would overmask** with this (very rare) true maximum conductive loss in the test ear.

Summary and Discussion of Masking Dilemmas for Spondee Threshold

The "Down 20 rule" works most times – the common exception is NTE significant conductive loss, where undermasking can occur. TE conductive loss can cause the "Down 20" rule to have problems, but you would need a near true maximum conductive loss before overmasking becomes a concern. The "Down 20" formula is simple (and therefore less prone to error) so it is recommended for the "plain vanilla" cases of asymmetrical sensorineural hearing loss, which is what you see most often in most clinical situations.

To review, if you have NTE conductive loss, then "Down 20" can undermask. Base your calculations on Minimum Masking Levels: go above that.

If the test ear has conductive loss, double check. Calculate MMax and make sure that it is below your "Down 20" level is below MMax. The test ear conductive loss has to be very large before overmasking becomes a concern when obtaining a spondee threshold.

If you have significant bilateral conductive loss, you will need to carefully calculate minimum and maximum. Similar to pure-tone testing with bilateral conductive loss, a masking dilemma may occur when trying to obtain the spondee threshold.

Example Spondee Threshold Masking Dilemma

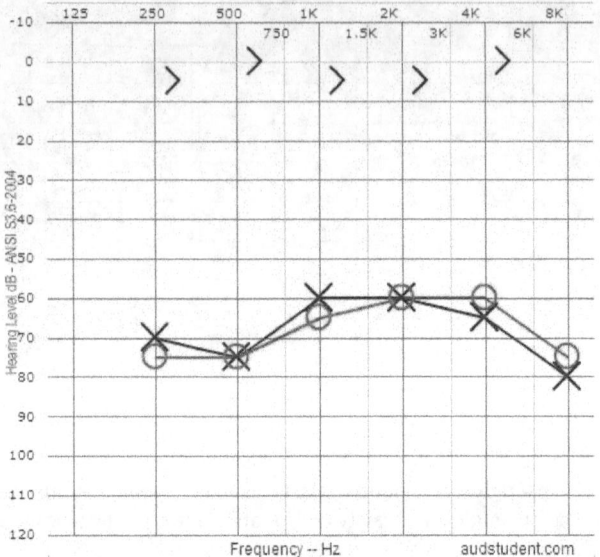

Figure 10-10. Classic masking dilemma audiogram. It appears there is bilateral conductive loss. If you were to attempt to (plateau) mask the pure-tone results, you would have the erroneous finding of two dead ears. Consider what you would do if you did NOT yet have bone-conduction thresholds, but assume from immittance and patient report that the loss is conductive, most likely bilaterally. Let's examine the left ear. I expect a ~65 dB HL unmasked spondee threshold. Can I mask to find that threshold, if it is truly the left ear threshold? (Perhaps the left ear is dead, and I'm measuring crossover from presenting to the left ear, but stimulating the right cochlea.)

The **Minimum Masking** formula = estimated spondee threshold (65) – IA (60) + 10 (in case the spondee threshold is a bit higher than I guessed) + NTE biggest ABG from 500-8k Hz (75 dB) = **90 dB HL.**

The **Maximum Masking Level** = best bone (0 dB HL) + 55 dB HL = **55 dB EM.** This defines the **masking dilemma:** I need a minimum of 90 but I will potentially overmask with 55 dB EM. If the loss were less severe, for spondee threshold testing (not for word recognition), you could try to plateau mask. Note that the **Down 20** rule, if the loss is bilaterally conductive, would be 65 estimated spondee threshold – 20 = **45 dB EM.** The "Down 20" rule undermasks dramatically. The 45 dB EM is not even audible!

Word Recognition Testing

Recognizing the Need for Masking

Although you need to mask for word recognition testing more often than for spondee threshold testing, at least you know the presentation level since you choose it! That eliminates that ambiguity you had with spondee threshold testing (what if it comes in a bit worse than I guessed?) To determine the need for masking, take the level of speech you plan to use for word recognition testing, subtract 60 dB. If there is any reason to believe that the non-test ear bone-conduction thresholds (in the 500 to 8k Hz range) are lower than that, then mask.

Formula for Min Masking: Word Recognition Testing Presentation Level – 50 dB + Largest Significant NTE ABG (500 to 8k Hz)

The minimum masking formula changes from what is used for spondee threshold testing. With spondee testing, you entertained the possibility of the spondee threshold coming in a bit higher than your best guess, and adjusted the masking level to account for that. You don't do that for word recognition testing, since you know exactly the level you will use when testing, so the formula is presentation level – 60 dB IA + 10 dB pad + largest significant NTE air-bone gap (500 to 8k Hz) which simplifies to **presentation level – 50 dB + largest significant NTE air-bone gap (500 to 8k Hz).**

Formula for Max Mask: Best TE BC threshold from 500 to 8k Hz + 55 dB

The maximum masking formula is the same as for spondee threshold testing: Find the best estimated bone-conduction threshold (and guess low rather than high to be safe, you don't want to overmask). Add 55 dB. While this is the "ideal" maximum, a little bit of crossback isn't going to lower the test ear word recognition score. If you can avoid going above MMax, please do so, but if the crossback is well below the perceived loudness of the speech signal, then it will not lower the word recognition score. We will examine this idea further below.

The "Down 20" Formula

The simple "Down 20" formula remains simple: Subtract 20 from the presentation level. As with spondee threshold testing, this formula risks undermasking with NTE conductive loss, and overmasking with TE conductive loss, but as we will explore further below, the overmasking probably won't interfere with understanding the monosyllabic words presented to the test ear.

Word Recognition Examples
Asymmetrical Sensorineural Hearing Loss

As with spondee threshold testing, the "Down 20" formula works well for word recognition testing. See Figure 10-11.

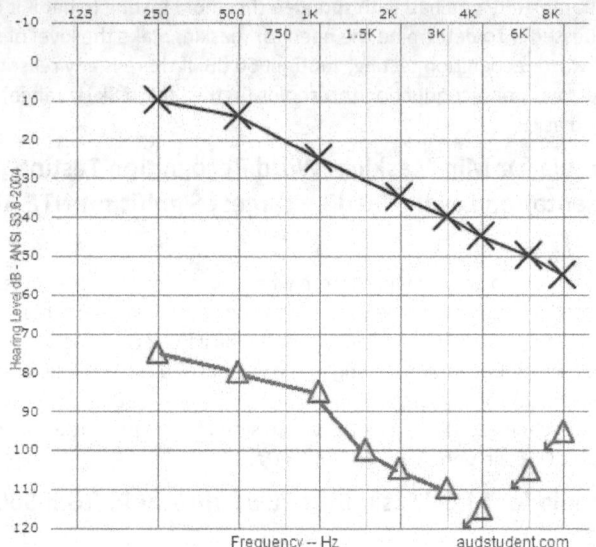

Figure 10-11. This case assumed sensorineural loss bilaterally. Choosing the level for word recognition is challenging. To ensure audibility, I'd like to test at 120 dB HL, but that might be uncomfortable for the patient. Let's assume the patient can tolerate that level, at least for a 25-word list, and that the audiometer is capable of producing that output level.

The **minimum masking level** = 120 – 60 IA + 10 pad = **70 dB EM.**

(The formula simplifies to 120 – 50 = 70 dB EM.)

The **maximum masking level** is theoretically 70 dB HL 500 Hz threshold (in case there is an insignificant 10 dB conductive overlay at 500 Hz) plus 55 dB: **125 dB EM.**

Down 20 recommends **100 dB EM**. Again, for this bilateral sensorineural loss the Down 20 formula recommendation is in between minimum and maximum. We have the "Goldilocks" level – not too loud, not too quiet, just right. What's not to love about this simple formula? Conductive loss, see next figures.

NTE Conductive Loss Word Recognition Example

As was true for spondee threshold testing, conductive loss in the NTE requires higher masking levels, and the "Down 20" rule can undermask.

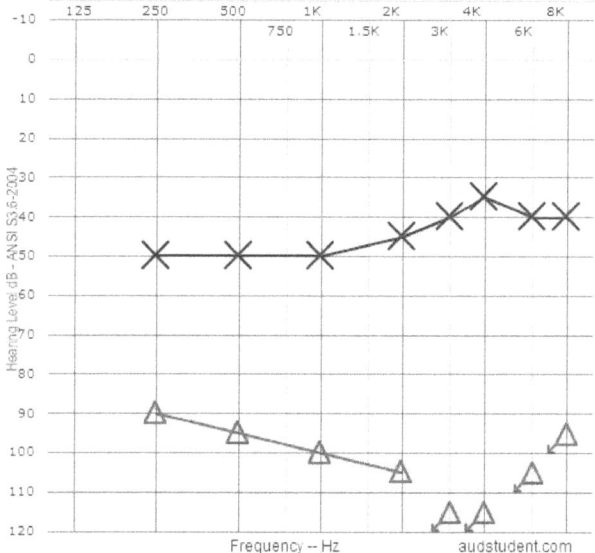

Figure 10-12. This is a case of left ear **(NTE ear) conductive loss.** Again, let's assume the patient can tolerate 120 dB HL word recognition testing.

Min Mask = 120 - 50 + largest NTE ABG of 50 dB = **120 dB EM.**

The right ear was assumed to have sensorineural loss. **Max Mask** = best realistic bone at 500 Hz and above, and we will again consider that it's possible that there may be a small conductive overlay. Use 85 as the best reasonably possible 500 Hz bone-conduction threshold, add 55. Yazza. If you were able to produce **140 dB EM** in the left ear, that would still not be problematic – it would not overmask.

So, how does the "Down 20" rule fair? Not well. But you know that already – NTE conductive loss attenuates the masking noise and can lead to undermasking. Here, the **Down 20** rule says 120 presentation level – 20 = **100 dB HL**, but the minimum needed was 120 dB EM. That is **insufficient masking noise.**

Test Ear Conductive Loss Word Recognition Testing Examples

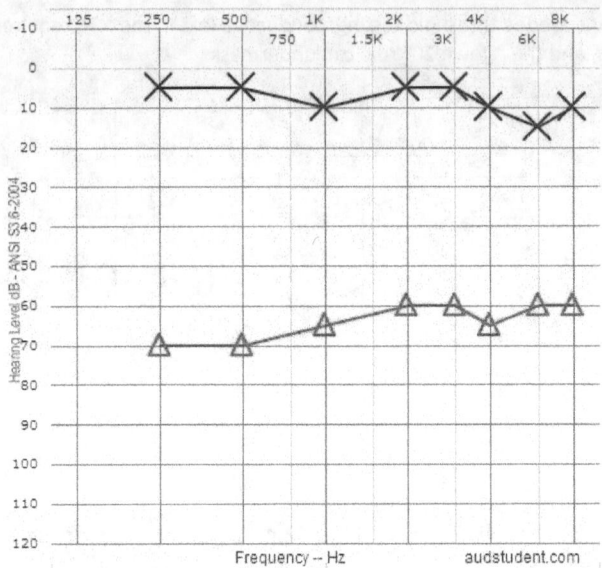

Figure 10-13. The right ear loss is presumed to be conductive based on immittance testing. Since conductive losses don't have recruitment, I would like to test word recognition at 30-40 dB sensation level. Let's assume that the patient finds 100 dB HL speech comfortable.

Min Mask = 100 – 50 (-60 IA plus the 10 dB pad) = **50 dB EM**

Potentially one may find a 0 or 5 dB BC threshold for the right ear, so **Max Mask = 55/60**.

Down 20 rule indicates that we would use **80 dB EM** and that has a potential to cause problems. The crossback that could be as much as 20 dB, and that might start to interfere with speech understanding. (The signal is at about 35 dB sensation level, so the 20 dB of crossback probably would not cause a reduction in the word understanding score.)

Let's examine a larger test ear conductive loss next – see Figure 10-14.

Chapter 10. Speech Masking

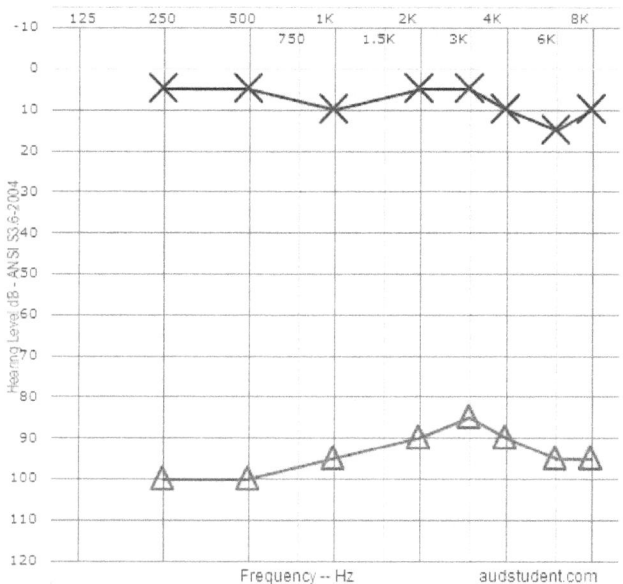

Figure 10-14. Let's make the right ear conductive loss extreme and do the calculations using the maximum output of the audiometer, 125 dB HL.

Min Mask = 125-50 = **75 dB EM**.

Max Mask will remain at **50/55 dB EM** since we are assuming that the loss in the right ear is conductive. We know we have to use that 75 dB EM, so let's think more about the consequences of this overmasking. If the interaural attenuation is 60 dB (remember, most people will have greater IA values), then the crossed back noise level at the test ear cochlea is 15 dB EM. If the spondee threshold had been 95 dB HL, this means the 125 dB HL word recognition stimuli are presented at 30 dB SL. The signal-to-noise ratio is still favorable (I consider above 10 dB favorable). The patient should be able to understand 30 dB sensation level test words even with 15 dB SL crossback at the same cochlea, so I would feel comfortable using the 75 dB EM minimum masking level.

Here the Down 20 formula really doesn't work: it overmasks. The recommended 105 dB EM could cross back as 45 dB EM in the test ear cochlea, which could eliminate the hearing of the 30 dB sensation level signal.

Some Crossback Doesn't Matter: Consider the Signal-to-Noise Ratio at the TE Cochlea

As the examples above have introduced, crossback isn't always "the end of the world." This concept applies for spondee threshold testing as well, but word recognition testing involves presenting supra-threshold level stimuli, requiring higher masking levels, and greater crossback levels are seen.

If some of the noise crosses BACK to the test ear cochlea, that can interfere with word recognition, but it does not necessarily do so. Examine Figure 10-15.

Chapter 10. Speech Masking

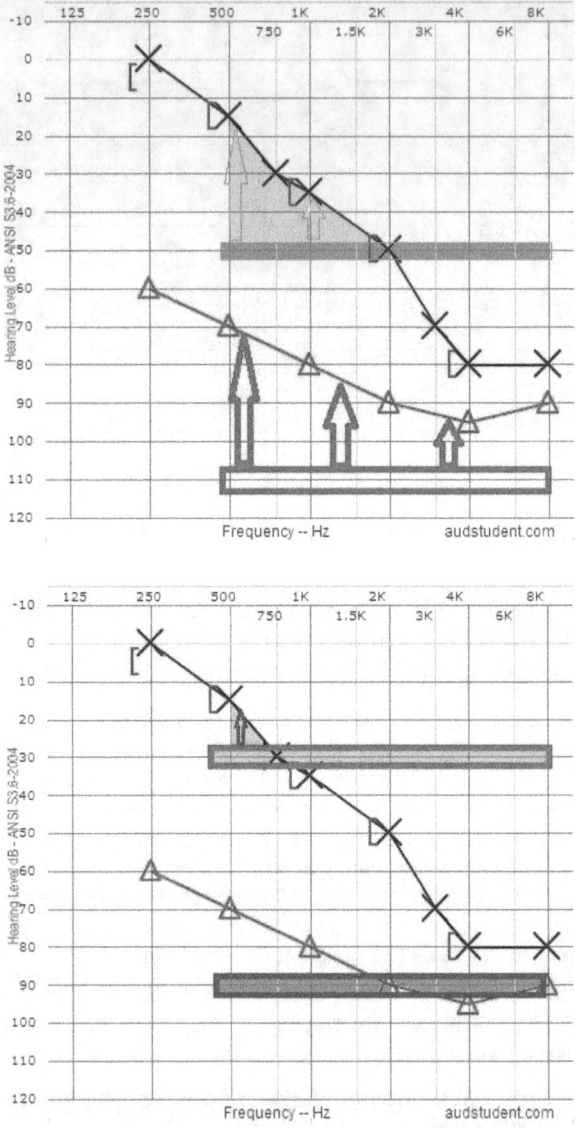

Figure 10-15. The right ear has a large conductive overlay. Word recognition testing is conducted at 110 dB HL. The crossover can be heard in the left ear. The minimum masking level = 110-50: 60 dB EM. The maximum masking level = 15+55 = 70. Using anything within that narrow range of 60 to 70 dB EM would be fine, but let's assume the audiologist was having an off day and used the "Down 20" formula, presenting 90 dB of noise to the left ear. As shown on the bottom of the figure, this could cause some crossback to the cochlea, which is audible at and below 750 Hz. Would it degrade word recognition performance? No, that's unlikely. The sensation level of the speech signal (dark, lower arrows on the top figure) is above the sensation level of the crossback (arrows on the bottom of the figure.)

Chapter 10. Speech Masking

Masking Dilemmas with Word Recognition Testing

It is possible to have a masking dilemma for word recognition testing – the same situation as creates a masking dilemma for pure-tone testing: bilateral maximum or near maximum conductive loss. Refer to Figure 10-16.

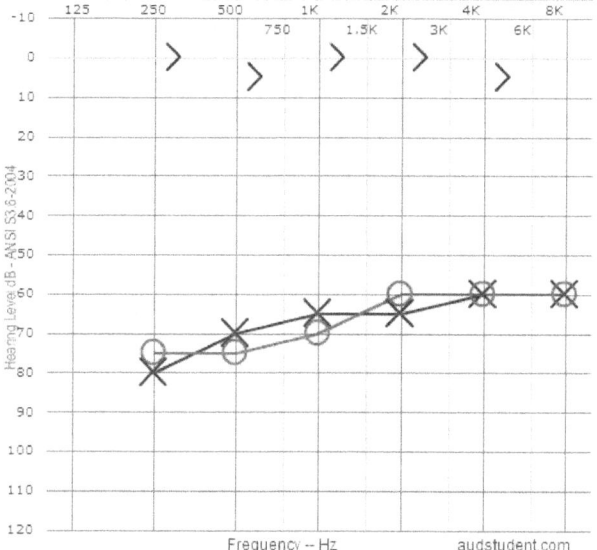

Figure 10-16. Immittance test results are consistent with bilateral conductive loss: pure-tone testing with masking presents with a masking dilemma. So will spondee threshold and word recognition testing. Assume that you test left ear word recognition at 100 dB HL, which will be about 30 dB sensation level. The minimum masking level = 100-50+largest NTE ABG (about 70 dB) = 120. The crossback level (120-60) = 60. Since the loss is conductive, that means that the crossback is at about 60 dB sensation level. The noise that crosses back to the test ear cochlea will be louder than the speech sensation level (30 dB SL). The person won't hear the words, let alone be able to repeat them. You'll have the same problem with finding the spondee threshold. If the left ear spondee comes in at 65 dB HL, our formula recommends to use (65-40+~70) at minimum 95 dB EM, which could crossback at 35 dB EM, which will prevent hearing. (Remember, the cochlea does the speech recognition – the level of speech reaching the cochlea after attenuation by the conductive loss is about 0 dB HL. The crossback of 35 is more than enough to prevent you from measuring a 70 dB spondee threshold.) What would happen? You would find an spondee threshold perhaps of 40 dB HL instead – elevated by the crossback. Then you would recognize that you aren't using enough masking noise since the spondee threshold was not what was expected. You'd increase the noise – and that would cause more overmasking, elevating the spondee threshold further.

Reporting on Results Influenced by Overmasking

When you have a potential masking dilemma, my recommendation is to calculate your minimum and maximum levels. If your minimum is above the maximum, think about the amount of crossback that could be created when you use that minimum level – and think about it frequency by frequency. Compare the crossback to the sensation level of the stimulus. If your sensation level is higher than the crossback by 10 dB or more, then the crossback likely has little or no effect

If there is more crossback, e.g. crossback is at 30 dB above the bone-conduction thresholds of the test ear, and the word recognition signal is 35 dB above the air-conduction thresholds, then the word recognition score is probably lowered. This is particularly true for those with sensorineural loss – their word recognition scores are lowered in the presence of competing signals. If you cannot lower the noise without undermasking, then I suggest that you make a note in your report, e.g. "Contralateral masking noise crossback potentially lowered the word recognition score." You could also test unmasked and note "Because of the masking difficulties/dilemma potentially reducing the word recognition score, unmasked testing was conducted, but is influenced by the non-test ear participation. True word recognition performance is likely in the range between the masked and unmasked scores."

Summary of Speech Masking Concepts (Insert Earphone Use)

Need for Masking

When masking for speech, particularly word recognition testing, you must be vigilant about the need to mask. Remember to determine if the signal level – 60 dB is above the NTE best bone-conduction threshold (in the range of 500 to 8000 Hz). If so, masking is needed.

"Down 20" Formula is Ideal for Sensorineural Hearing Loss, Generally Adequate for Test Ear Conductive Loss, but Undermasks Significant NTE Conductive Loss Cases

Stay away from the simple "stimulus level – 20" rule if the non-test ear is conductive. It works wonderfully for sensorineural losses, and is simple to use. When the test ear has conductive loss, consider whether the crossback might interfere. (Noise level – 60: is that significantly above the TE bone-conduction thresholds? If so, determine the stimulus sensation level. You are still OK if the stimulus is at least 10 dB above the crossback level.) Be very careful with significant NTE conductive loss, there it is better to use the minimum masking formula. The Down 20 rule tends to cause undermasking with NTE conductive components

Minimum Masking Formula: Expected Spondee Threshold – 40 + Largest NTE ABG; Word Recognition Testing Level – 50 + Largest NTE ABG

We want to avoid having to raise the masking noise if the spondee threshold is slightly higher than predicted. Take your best estimate of the spondee threshold and adjust the formula by 10 dB more, in case the spondee threshold is a bit higher than your guess, which gives us the formula **Minimum Level = Expected Spondee Threshold – 40 + Largest Significant NTE Air-Bone Gap (500 to 8k Hz).**

For word recognition testing, you know precisely what the stimulus intensity is, so the formula is **Minimum Level = Expected Spondee Threshold – 50 + Largest Significant NTE Air-Bone Gap (500 to 8k Hz).**

MMax is the Same for Word Recognition and Spondee Testing, but You Don't Care about Minor Overmasking, Especially with Word Recognition Testing

Since the minimum speech IA is 60 dB, the maximum masking level formula is **Max Mask = Best Test Ear Bone-Conduction Threshold (500 to 8k Hz) + 55 dB**. If you want to be conservative, you can lower your estimate of the bone-conduction threshold by 10 dB (in case there are minor air-bone gaps).

Remember that some crossback and overmasking may not be a problem, especially with sloping losses. If the crossback is only audible in the lowest frequencies, then even for spondee threshold testing, the results may not be invalidated. With word recognition testing, you are presenting at a level that is suprathreshold. If the crossback is well below the level of the speech at the test ear cochlea, then the crossback doesn't affect the word recognition score much if at all. Ideally, you would examine the sensation level of the noise above the test ear bone-conduction thresholds. Compare to the sensation level of the speech above the test ear air-conduction thresholds. You would want the speech sensation level to be at a minimum 10 dB louder. If undermasking problems prevent you from lowering the speech level when this criterion is not met, document that the word recognition scores may be lowered due to overmasking.

References:

- Cox, R.M. & Moore, J.N. (1988). Composite speech spectrum for hearing aid gain prescriptions. *Journal of Speech and Hearing Research, 31,* 102-107.
- Sklare, D.A., & Denenberg, L.J. (1987). Interaural attenuation for Tubephone™ insert earphones. *Ear and Hearing, 8*(5), 298-300

www.ingramcontent.com/pod-product-compliance
Lightning Source LLC
Chambersburg PA
CBHW070246190526
45169CB00001B/316